TABLE LESSONS:

Insights in the Practice of Massage Therapy

DOUGLAS NELSON

ISBN: 0615445608
ISBN-13: 9780615445601

This book is dedicated to two very special clients, Clara and Margit, who patiently mentored a young and uneducated therapist to reason and question. While both are now deceased, the legacy of their wisdom is alive in every story in this book.

FOREWORD

For anyone who has had the pleasure of being witness to the teaching, the treating or the writing of Douglas Nelson, the word that immediately springs forth is elegance. Having personally had experience with all of these facets and the mastery within which he commands them, it is nothing less than true privilege to have access in such a format to him. It is rare to find such greatness in any of the above listed qualities, but to have excellence in all is even more unfound in any profession.

Within these pages, Nelson sets out to accomplish a simple yet profound task: to tell through story necessary and essential clinical insights and principles relevant to massage therapy and specifically that of his own stamp of work, Precision Neuromuscular Therapy (PNMT). To those unacquainted with PNMT, it is much more than mere rote procedure and has very little in common with the older work derived from Raymond Nimmo's Receptor Tonus method and what later became in the massage world known as Neuromuscular Therapy. It is and has become more of an approach than a technique. Problem solving using the hands encapsulates PNMT in a nutshell. Nelson pulls from such varied fields and influences such as the Trigger Point work of Kellgren, Travell and Simons, functional and dynamic anatomical approaches, applicable structural methodology, exclusionary and orthopedic evaluation, and most of all, current neurophysiologic understanding of the mechanisms of neuromusculoskeletal pain and dysfunction. Douglas utilizes the most effective methods based on the latest research and his vast clinical experience rather than dogma and passed down routine. PNMT is again, first and foremost about solving problems that our patients present to us every day.

When someone enters our therapy office with presenting symptoms of low back pain (LBP), how do we know where to begin, what to do and what not to? The answers to these questions are at the heart of PNMT. There is no LBP routine; there is only that particular patient and the process of determining what structures and mechanisms are relevant to their pain on that day. The understanding of what manual method to use flows from the process of deduction during the patient evaluation. Constant reassessment insures that our interventions are either well-conceived or in need of redirection. In PNMT, every second demands the utmost concentration and skill from the practitioner. The success of our clinical effort is in direct relationship to the therapist's depth of understanding of the complex interactions and interventions of the somatic system.

To learn and execute at the apex of any skilled trade there are a few paths and strategies one can take. The most common and proven means of practice are the models of music, sports and chess.

The music model relies on rehearsal and an incredibly high number of repetitions. We all do this to a greater or lesser extent with our anatomy, physiology and hands-on training as therapists. We repeat techniques and reread information.

The sports model consists of conditioning in a general way that will be important to our craft and then in a more specific way to critical and specific skills to the trade. In massage this may consist of doing maintenance exercises to our hands and bodies to ensure that we remain healthy in order to give our careers longevity.

The last approach is the chess model. The famed and late physiotherapist Geoff Maitland gave a great analogy of this model's relevance to manual therapy when he said, "it is like a game of chess where different 'pieces' can be moved in many different ways, and where plans are made and destroyed and changed until the goal is achieved." The chess model is also known in different fields as the case method. This type of directly applicable theorization of 'putting oneself in the a situation' and laying out all the possible ways one would react and progress through the scenario given is vital to the actual process that occurs in therapy sessions. To be given a case study and work your way through it forces you to apply all of your training and acquired skills in order to 'play out' what and how you would do what you do. The limitation of this method as described so far is that you are at the threshold of your own understandings and capabilities. In order to improve, for instance in the game of chess, you learn from what the grand masters have done in similar situations. Their expertise has been honed and developed from years of intense deliberate practice and study. In other words, in order to become better you must learn and study with those who are beyond your present clinical capacities.

Douglas Nelson embodies this 'grand master' of the game of manual therapy. To be able to glean awareness from such a 'Delphi' of the field can only improve one's own skills. Reading the cases within this book places you at the foot of this consummate clinician. Certain insights can only be harvested through direct experience as is conducted by Nelson at his clinic in Champaign, where he invites therapists from around the country into his treatment room to learn by watching him conduct and orchestrate sessions with clients who suffer with varied painful ailments. There is no replacement for such an encounter with clinical adroitness. However, there is one major advantage to learning by means of the medical tales that Douglas spins here; that is one of elapsed time and reflection. When observing him in real time at his clinic one can only see the 'chess moves' that occurred during that place in the game of patient care. You don't get to hear how the patient progressed days and weeks later. You don't get to hear the interpretation and conclusions based on their progress from a master clinician's point of view. Here in lies the great advantage of absorbing yourself in a book such as this.

The worth of this book is measured far beyond the simple and typical accounts of success after success in patient interactions. If you do what you know and it works, there is very little development and growth as a practitioner. Unfortunately, what will often jettison clinical understanding are the failures that occur during patient care and how we react when we encounter a similar situation in the future. Furthermore, working with actual patients is less about going in with a great strategy and following that course, but rather knowing one's own limitations and competently handling such positions. This book takes you through all these crucial steps from initial "strategy", "failing and learning," "differential assessment" and finally patient practitioner "communication." All of these steps are vital to the craft and art of manual therapy. I hope that you take heed to read, contemplate, reflect and apply the principles that lie here within to your own practice as the book was intended. In so doing you will surely be doing a great service to your own advancement as a clinician as well as the service that will follow to the patients that you serve.

Seth Will

TABLE OF CONTENTS

INTRODUCTION

Praxis: the translation of principles or ideas into practice. I, who love words, have loved the word praxis from the moment I first heard it. What I find so powerful is that a single word represents such an important and encompassing endeavor. As a clinician and teacher, I have spent much time reflecting on how best to convey my clinical insights and experience so that others may benefit. Some lessons, however simple, have taken me far too long to fully realize their importance. As a teacher, I often wonder how to best convey this knowledge so that others will not have to repeat my mistakes.

Over time, I have gravitated to using stories from my experiences in the clinic to illustrate strategy and assessment skills. Stories have power that mere principles do not; they give meaning and context to information we might otherwise overlook. I often hear my students repeat a story I told them years ago, stories that I do not even remember. The principle embedded in the story is not forgotten, but forever embodied in the narrative itself. The story represents praxis, translating knowledge into practice.

For those of us who do manual therapy, each client is a story of its own. Manual therapy is unique in the amount of time spent in close relationship between therapist and client. It is a microcosm of relationship; a back and forth of learning, listening, perception, and action. The goal of the relationship is to produce a desired outcome, typically a decrease in physical discomfort. The tighter the goal sought, the more difficult that goal is to achieve. There are multiple ways to maximize effectiveness, just as there are a myriad of ways to veer off track. Therapists learn to be more effective by benefiting either from their own experience or the shared experience of others.

I have taught the principles of manual therapy skills to thousands of therapists in multiple therapeutic disciplines. Some of these principles were taught to me by my own instructors and others I have learned through struggle and experience. It gives me great pleasure to share an insight which took me many years to discover, knowing that I can expedite another person's learning and effectiveness.

Many of these concepts and principles are simple yet profound. These stories are part of my personal history in the clinic, part of the fabric that is my professional life. While I learn much from study and from my own mentors, it is often the clients that grace my treatment table who teach me and motivate me to keep learning. They inspire me to keep learning and growing both personally and professionally.

Douglas Nelson

SECTION ONE: STRATEGY

When people ask me to define Precision Neuromuscular Therapy (PNMT), I often explain that PNMT is a problem solving manual therapy approach for soft-tissue pain and discomfort. While this seems simple, it took me a long time to get clear about what I am teaching and why.

One of the most pivotal moments came in a discussion I had with Sandy Fritz, a wonderful therapist and educator in the field of massage therapy. When I described my struggle with defining PNMT, it was Sandy who clarified it for me:

"Your problem is, in a field where everyone else is teaching technique, you are teaching a way of thinking and problem solving."

Ever since that moment, the focus of the seminars has been helping participants master effective problem solving strategies. The sources of strategies are legion; so many different disciplines struggle with effective problem solving. I thoroughly enjoy chatting with my friends in other professions to hear how they strategize to tackle problems in their chosen field. No matter the discipline, we all wish to be as efficient and as effective as possible. In my experience, success is often a matter of the wisdom of the approach, not just the techniques executed. The following stories reflect various strategies to the administration of soft-tissue therapy.

WHERE IS THE DRAMA?

Ms. H came to the office with complaints of restriction of right rotation of the neck. Having heard that I deal only with specific challenges, she felt her neck met the criteria. She sat down at the side of my table and showed me her rotational abilities.

"It looks like your range is quite limited. Let's measure it to see how restricted it is. While we are at it, let's look at all your neck range of motion measurements. Before we do that, I have one question. When you turn your head to the right, where do you feel the tightness, on the left or on the right?"

"On the left," she said, pointing to her neck.

I took Ms. H through the complete range of cervical motion. Her right rotation was only 40 degrees; her left rotation was 70 degrees. Her lateral flexion to the right was also limited, 20 degrees less than lateral flexion to the left.

I tried rotating her head passively to the right, but as soon as I neared the motion barrier, she tensed in a protective spasm. Moving her head into right lateral flexion, it was clear that there was a great deal of tension in the lateral flexors on the left, but no protective spasm. Therein was the opening I needed.

Slowly, I began to address each of the muscles that create lateral flexion to the left. As I examined the tissue, she was surprised at how tender these muscles on the left were, since she had been totally focused on the right side.

"That is surprisingly tender, but what I really struggle with is this," she said, demonstrating right rotation. Catching her head before she could turn her head fully to the right, I nodded in approval. I could tell she was a bit perplexed at why I wasn't dealing with trying to increase her right rotation.

"I understand that we need to increase your right rotation, and I will address it soon. Right now, I need to set the stage by diffusing the tenderness on the left side."

"It is certainly tender, but wait until you feel the right side," she stated. "If the left side is that bad, the right side must be terrible."

Slowly, the session progressed in this fashion. I carefully and thoroughly released muscles that create left lateral flexion. Periodically, I would gently check right rotation, stopping at the very first sign of restriction. Just before Ms. H could redirect me to address the right side, I would return to treating muscles on the left side. Each time I subtly checked right rotation, it was a little less volatile and hypersensitive. I tried to do these measurements without drawing much attention to it, fearful that she would once again to try to push me to attack her right side with a vengeance.

Picking up her head, I carefully moved it into right and left lateral flexion. She was remarkably good at letting me move her neck passively. Sensing a little more stiffness flexing her neck to the right, I then had her raise her left arm and put it up near her head, which puts the levator scapula on a stretch. This markedly decreased lateral flexion to the right, implicating the levator scapula as a major source of her restriction. After treating the levator scapula, flexion to the right was far better.

"Should we start working on my rotation now? I don't know how much time is left, but I want you to spend the rest of the time on that."

"Sure. Why don't you sit up and let's take a look at what we have left to do?"

As she tried right rotation of her neck again, I relished the look on her face when she turned to full range. In disbelief, she brought her head back neutral and tried turning again. Not accepting what she felt, she tried a third time, turning her head with even more ease.

Ms. H sat up and looked at me in disbelief.

"What just happened here?" she asked with astonishment.

"Where is the drama, the pain, the sacrifice?" she inquired with this wonderful, sarcastic grin on her face.

"I think I can arrange more drama, along with some suffering and sacrifice, if you think that would help," I replied.

"Okay, seriously. I do not understand how that was possible. I have been waiting for 40 minutes for you to address the source of my pain, and now it is gone without seemingly even treating it. That seems like magic," she said shaking her head in disbelief.

"It is anything but magical. In the neck, rotation to the right is also accompanied by lateral flexion to the right. If you remember, your right lateral flexion was quite limited in relation to the left. The muscles on the left side of your neck that stopped you from laterally flexing right were also players in limiting your rotation to the right. When I improved one range, I affected the other."

"It just isn't the battle I thought we would be fighting," she said, still rotating her head to the right in disbelief.

"Sometimes, you can win the war without fighting a battle at all," I couldn't resist retorting.

"Touché!" she responded.

EITHER WAY, YOU WIN

The act of washing hands. Such a simple thing and yet one would be amazed at the number of times this little discipline has led to all manner of outcomes in my office. I suppose it is the nature of any community; the members gather around a central place which is functionally oriented. The agoras in ancient Greece, the water cooler at an office, or guests at a dinner party are great examples of this. Invite people over for dinner and observe the traffic pattern. If your house has 5,000 square feet and four floors, the guests still congregate in the kitchen, no matter how hard you try to entice them elsewhere. In my office setting, the center of the vortex seems to be the sink.

One of the things I enjoy most about having a large group practice of massage therapists is the collaboration with each other on difficult cases. We do not have a formal process for discussing these sorts of things; I tried that and it failed miserably. Some topics emerge much better spontaneously than when formally scheduled. On this day, while washing my hands, another interesting case was about to unfold.

"You will love this; I think I have a client with bilateral frozen shoulder."

Mike tossed out this little salvo as I was lost in soap and water; I glanced back to see his face. Mike is a seriously bright guy and a great therapist who also has a mischievous sense of humor. I never know if he is serious or just yanking my chain.

"Bilateral?" I repeated.

"Yep, bilateral," Mike asserted. "She is a great lady, probably in her mid-forties and back in graduate school. This started about two months ago. Would you like to see her with me?"

I agreed and the client was very open to having both of us assess her shoulders. We met about two weeks later and Mike gave me all the previous notes to read over. I glanced at them, but tried to gather facts about her condition without drawing conclusions. I find that I am unconsciously swayed by another person's conclusions as to the nature of the problem.

Ms. D was indeed a charming and obviously brilliant woman; the kind of client I really enjoy seeing. With a client who is this bright, I tend to verbalize every part of the deductive process. This is certainly not true for all clients; some clients don't want to know anything but the final answer and others get a little uncomfortable with the process. Ms. D is my ideal client; one who can participate fully in the process.

"It started about two months ago, the pain came in sharp electric stabs if I moved incorrectly. There is no precipitating event I can ascribe the pain to, it just slowly came on. First, it was these random catches, but then it started to take a different form. It seems like these catches are getting closer together and I am losing mobility in my shoulders. There are times though, when it seems OK. "

"This happened to both shoulders at the same time?" I asked.

"Well, it started with the left but quickly moved to the right. I am not sure which is worse at this point."

I had Ms. D show me her forward flexion and abduction range of motion, neither of which were normal but neither was the 50% limitation typical of frozen shoulder. I had Ms. D lie supine on the table and examined her internal and external range of motion. This was essentially the same; limited, but not severely limited. More interestingly, she would ratchet her way through the whole process; I could feel the muscles catching and letting go in an uneven way. As the muscles would 'catch', she would almost respond as in pain, but then the muscle would let go again. This process continued until we got closer to the real end of range, which was about fifty degrees of external rotation of the humerus and 25 degrees of internal rotation.

"Do you notice anything else, other muscular issues?" I inquired.

"My calves have been really tight, especially when I awaken. I do not sleep very well at all. My sleep is very choppy. I often wake up, mostly because my left shoulder hurts."

"My goal for today is to figure out whether this is in the frozen shoulder arena or possibly something else. What you described is classic for frozen shoulder, so let's score one point in that category."

At that point, Mike interjected. "But her range wasn't that restricted."

"True, but this could easily be stage one frozen shoulder. In stage one, range isn't limited yet but there are often episodic shooting pains. Most important is the presence of nocturnal pain, which is a hallmark of frozen shoulder syndrome."

"What about the leg pain? Is that connected?" asked Ms. D.

"Good point, I replied. "That does not fit in the frozen shoulder model, so score a point for some unknown problem. By unknown, I am referring to some chemical source of irritation, rather than mechanical."

"What exactly do you mean by that?" asked Ms. D.

"Mechanical pain is pain that is made better or worse with movement or position. If you strain a muscle in your back, it is made worse with and action that stretches it or makes it contract. Plus, you can position yourself, at least temporarily, in a way that relieves it. A chemical source of irritation, like inflammation, is different. Think of a bladder or kidney infection. No position or activity makes it better."

"Do you think this is mechanical or chemical?"

"That is exactly the issue I am trying to address. Unfortunately, you present symptoms of both."

"What about the shooting pains in my left arm and bicep area?"

"That is absolutely classic for stage one frozen shoulder. In fact, it is why so many stage one frozen shoulders are misdiagnosed as bicipital tendonitis. Generally, it gets treated as a tendonitis and that doesn't help at all. As the frozen shoulder progresses, the patient gradually keeps losing range of motion. By the time he/she has gone to a different doctor for help, the frozen shoulder has progressed to stage two, which is easy to diagnose. That second or third doctor probably wonders how in the world the first doctor could have blown such an easy call. In reality, they are probably misdiagnosing the stage one frozen shoulder patients they are seeing now."

"Wow, is frozen shoulder that little understood?"

"You bet; there is a lack of understanding about the condition and worse yet, a lot of misinformation out there. Success rates for therapy are pretty underwhelming and no one really understands what causes frozen shoulder in the first place. Anything else of note medically? Diabetes? Thyroid issues?"

"Umm, my doctor just ran a thyroid test and I was low. I am not diabetic. Why do you ask?"

"These symptoms can be part of a thyroid deficiency; there is some evidence that a thyroid deficiency can also be linked to frozen shoulder onset. The same is true for diabetes; frozen shoulder is far more prevalent in diabetics."

"Why am I so sore here?" Ms. D asked while pointing to her upper trapezius.

"Lifting your arms out to the side, the movement you have the most trouble with, is both a movement of the arm and also the shoulderblade. Since you can't lift your arm normally, that muscle that hurts you, the upper trapezius, overworks to help lift your arm out to the side. It is compensating for what you cannot do. If this is frozen shoulder, that muscle is in for a lot more work."

"Do you think this is frozen shoulder? From what you have said, a lot of what I report is leaning in that direction."

"A lot, but not all. It doesn't explain your leg pain and the stiffness you feel in the morning. The thing that is really bugging me is that it is bilateral. When Mike called me in, I was all set to shoot down the frozen shoulder idea because the odds of getting it on both sides at once are incredibly low. It isn't impossible, but I have to think that there must be some other reason, more chemical, that could account for all the symptoms you experience."

"Like what other things?" Ms. D wanted to know.

"This is where my knowledge ends. What I do know is that all those possibilities are the providence of your doctor. She sounds like a very bright and knowledgeable lady. I think this condition may be in her arena, not ours."

"She is great, but I have to say that she sounded just as perplexed as you do. She isn't sure what the cause is and is digging through the literature looking for a possible explanation."

"You should consider yourself lucky to have a doctor who isn't quick to come to a diagnosis. The fact that she is combing the literature is wonderful. You are in great hands."

"I am not sure she understands frozen shoulder with the same depth you do. I am anxious to relay to her what you have told me, I think it might explain a lot. Even though the odds are low, it seems like the best explanation so far."

I listened to Ms. D and thought about how lucky she was to have a doctor who was clearly providing thoughtful and reasoned care. I was just about to ask Ms. D if she would like me to talk to her doctor when a better strategy came to mind.

"Come to think of it, I have a better plan, if you are up for it. You are correct, the frozen shoulder criteria seems like the best explanation so far. It is possible that these other symptoms are not relevant to the real diagnosis, but what if they are? If your doctor is that open, and similarly perplexed, I am afraid that she too might agree that the best explanation for your pain is frozen shoulder syndrome."

"What's wrong with that, if I really do have frozen shoulder?"

"Nothing, except what if you don't? What if there is some underlying disease process that accounts for all these symptoms?

If your doctor buys my assessment, she will stop looking for other causes. That might be a really bad decision.

Here is another way to think of it. If it is frozen shoulder, we have tons of experience with it and can help you through the process. On the medical side, the success rate for most of the interventions isn't very promising. On our side, if it really is frozen shoulder, we can help speed up the road to recovery. On the other hand, if it isn't frozen shoulder and we treat it, it will delay you getting the correct diagnosis. I don't want you to come here for two months or more without progress, only to find out the problem is not frozen shoulder.

On the other hand, if she looks for a chemical solution while we address possible frozen shoulder issues, you have both bases covered. One of us will be wrong, but one of us will be right. Either way, you win. I am suggesting that you not relay my assessment to her because I am afraid she will think I am correct. Most importantly, nothing that we do will conflict with what your doctor will do. You have two therapeutic strategies, neither conflict with the other, but only one is right. It's perfect."

What followed was a bit of silence while everyone digested the plan. Each of us looked away, weighing the pluses and looking for minuses, and not really finding any. After a moment, we all looked at each other and three people broke out in a collective smile that confirmed we had just agreed on a plan. If it really was frozen shoulder, we had it covered. If it was a serious chemical imbalance or disease process, the doctor had it covered. Most importantly, all the bases were covered. Ms. D could not lose, she could only win.

Addendum: One of the most common reasons for poor medical care is an error in logic called confirmation bias. Doctors (and all health care providers) tend to look for information that confirms their preconceptions and thus ignore information that would refute the diagnosis. Once a physician makes a diagnosis, subsequent time is spent confirming the validity of the decision made. Symptoms that do not fit the diagnosis are often ignored as outliers. This can lead to disaster.

Any health care provider is going to assess a condition with the bias of his/her discipline. An orthopedist will see the problem as osseous in nature; a neurologist will diagnose the same problem as a neural pathology. A chiropractor will state that the same symptom is entirely due to vertebral subluxation. The therapist who is trained in Eastern medicine might speak of an energy imbalance, while another therapist is positive the symptom is due to fascial restriction. We each have a lens that is very limited and colored with our own bias. We all need to be careful to protect the people we serve by not overreaching our boundaries. Soft-tissue treatment works well when soft-tissue *is* the source of the problem. The bigger question is this: How do we know definitively that soft tissue restriction is the source of the client's pain? Much of my own research and clinical practice these days is geared to answering that simple question.

THAT PLACE BEHIND THE STOVE

"It isn't that I cannot lift my arm. I can, but it just does not feel the same as the other side. When I raise my left arm, I just lift it. When I am lifting my right arm, it takes much more effort and there is a little discomfort."

Miss D stood facing me, alternately lifting her arms in forward flexion. Her face narrowed as she concentrated on the differences between the movements of her arms.

"Does it look different? Can you see a difference in the range between the two arms?" she asked.

"If there is a difference it is very slight, probably not worth measuring," I replied. "But range of motion is only one criterion in evaluating your movement. Range of motion is a quantitative assessment; something I can measure and assign a number to. Your perception about the ease of movement is called a qualitative assessment; it is no less valid. Can you show me where you feel discomfort at the end of range?"

Miss D pointed to the deltoid tuberosity area on her right arm.

"I feel it somewhere in here. I say 'somewhere' because I cannot find the exact spot, nor can the other massage therapist I visited previously. Everything in this area (the deltoid tuberosity) is tender, but no place is 'the spot'. Maybe the problem was much deeper than the other therapist was willing to go, but I thought she was digging into my arm pretty aggressively. If we go any deeper, I am afraid I will have bruises."

"I wouldn't worry about that," I replied. "I don't think the problem is centered there in the first place."

Miss D gave me that polite look one gives when you think the other person is out of his/her mind.

"What? You are suggesting that there isn't a problem here?" she said pointing to her deltoid.

"Perhaps not. Lift your arm again and let me watch the movement."

As she lifted her right arm in forward flexion, I observed that her deltoid was indeed working hard, harder than it should. Asking her to hold her arm slightly away from her side, I palpated the teres muscles with a pincer palpation.

"Holy crap," she exclaimed. "Wow, is that tender!"

As my pincer palpation moved from the teres to the latissimus, she grimaced in pain and looked at me in disbelief.

"What the heck? I don't get it. Those places are outrageously tender. What is going on here?"

Before I could formulate an answer, she jumped in.

"Okay, wait. Why don't I feel the pain there instead of my deltoid? If the underside of my arm is that tender, I should feel the pain there. Maybe I was just super-sensitive. Could you do that again?"

Carefully, I compressed the latissimus between my thumb and finger and again she winced.

"Try that on the other side," she suggested.

Compressing the latissimus and teres on the left side, it was slightly tender.

"Are you pressing as hard on that side?" she asked.

"Actually, I am pressing what I would suspect is twice as hard."

"That is amazing. The right side is clearly a problem. I just don't understand how something can hurt that much without me knowing about it."

"The answer to that question lies in the principle of **habituation**. Your brain is always asking three questions of every stimulus: What is it? What does it mean? What do I need to do?

At some point in the past, there was an injury to these muscles. The injury does not have to be debilitating, but it certainly compromised the tissue. What people think is that time heals all, that these tissue injuries will improve without treatment. In many cases, this is not true.

Because the injury is not changing, your brain has to make a choice. This discomfort coming from the underside of the arm has not changed in multiple days. As the brain evaluates the meaning of the pain, it is clear that the tissue injury is not a serious threat, as it is not getting worse. While the brain is not sure what the problem is, it is reasonably sure that no action is needed. Your brain then simply put the input from that area into the background as there are more important things to attend to in daily life. When I compress the tissue, I bring it to the foreground."

"You certainly do!" she exclaimed. "I have to say, I felt like that area of my shoulder was fine until you started poking around," she said with a twinkle in her eye.

"I promise you I did not put it there. Would you let me carefully examine the tissue to see what lurks behind the shadows?"

As Miss D was lying supine, I slowly and carefully examined the teres, latissimus, and infraspinatus. While the tissue was tender, I could tell by the look on her face that she felt like the treatment was a very good thing.

"This feels so good, so right. I had no idea this was there in the first place. It is like that place behind the stove."

I looked at her quizzically.

"You know, when you move your stove over and find gross stuff that has been there for who knows how long. While it is gross, removing that stuff and cleaning the area is a great feeling. The thought that this stuff had been back there is revolting, but the satisfaction of cleaning it is worth the effort. Treating this part of my shoulder feels the same; like stuff has been there for a long time without me knowing about it."

As she relaxed, I continued to examine the tissue. Over the next ten minutes, the sensitivity diminished substantially. This improvement was as obvious to her as it was to me. Asking her to stand, I had her repeat forward flexion of her right arm. As she did, I could see an astonished look on her face.

"Wow! That is amazing. I don't feel any discomfort at all in the deltoid now. We didn't even touch that area and it is totally fine. How is that possible?"

"The muscles that we were treating do the opposite motion. Forward flexion requires the muscles underneath the shoulder to lengthen so unimpeded movement may happen. If the muscles under your arm tighten, they make the deltoid work much harder to counteract the pull. Not only is the deltoid lifting the arm up against gravity, it is also pulling against stronger muscles on the other side of the equation. No wonder the deltoid is complaining; it is doing twice the work. The pain is gone because now the deltoid is just lifting the arm, not fighting the opposite muscles at the same time."

"Amazing," she exclaimed. "Time to move the stove back!"

Strategy without tactics is the slowest route to victory. Tactics without strategy is the noise before defeat.

Sun Tzu

FRED IS DEAD

"Counterinsurgency?" he queried? I stared at Mr. K is disbelief...

Mr. K had come to my office with complaints of back pain that had started about two weeks previous. He had been doing some pretty heavy weight-lifting, ramping up his routine significantly previous to the injury. He had been doing deadlifts with weights and also a significant amount of cleaning in his basement. He first noticed the back pain while lifting a heavy box and moving it onto a cart. The motion involved in moving the heavy box was essentially side-bending to the left.

Mr. K's pain was on the right side of his low back. My first task was to gather information as to the exact source of his pain. There were several options and the task was to reasonably eliminate them one by one. As always, one symptom, many possible causes. I asked Mr. K to sidebend to the right and then to the left for me. Sidebending to the right was not painful, but sidebending to the left was. As he sidebent left, he felt pain on the right side of his low back. Since sidebending away from the pain was problematic, it pointed to muscular issues on the right side of his low back.

At this point, I decided to palpate his musculature to assess it both statically and dynamically. To static pressure, there was a slightly different feel to the two sides of his back, the right being a bit less compliant (stiffer) than the left. This difference was slight enough that I am not sure I could have known this without some prior knowledge on my part. The real issue was revealed when I asked him to sit in front of me and slowly sidebend to the left while I palpated his Quadratus Lumborum muscle on the right. As soon as the Quadratus muscle started to lengthen, it responded with a sudden contraction. The muscle was hyper-reactive about any change in length. More clearly, this seemed to be centered at exactly one spot; the insertion of the quadratus lumborum at the L4 transverse process.

Perhaps in years past, I might have focused my treatment on the perceived epicenter of Mr. K's pain. Since I was confident that L4 was the source of his pain based on dynamic evaluation and the extreme hypersensitivity, I decided not to address the epicenter but diffuse it by treating surrounding areas.

In the past, if I made this decision not to address the epicenter, I always explained to the client what I was doing and why. Without explanation, the client may have the feeling that I was lost and/or am fishing around the tissue. This can be especially frustrating to the client; they know at one point during the assessment, I indeed pressed on the exact epicenter. In his/her estimation, I must not have recognized the importance of the aforementioned epicenter, because I am not directly addressing it. In these cases, I usually explain how direct interventions carry some risk of backlash. Usually, this has been a rather tough sell, as the client would often prefer I just go right after the most sensitive area. I often relay a piece of data I once read; in a study of 300 military battles, six frontal assaults resulted in victory. For whatever reason, I cannot say why, I did not explain my strategy to Mr. K. I said nothing and just kept working diligently on assessing and treating his muscles.

As I was addressing surrounding tissue, trying carefully to ameliorate every avenue that might affect the L4 attachment, Mr. K turned his head and asked, "Counterinsurgency?" I was stunned. Absolutely speechless. I just stared at him while a faint (albeit restrained) smile emerged on his face. Never has anyone, ever, actually understood what I was doing and why. The look on his face told me that he 'got' the whole strategy from the moment I found the epicenter and did not pursue it. I remember thinking it a bit odd that he acknowledged how L4 recreated his symptoms, but he did not protest when I promptly moved on.

At that moment, I remembered that I noticed a small insignia on his lapel when he arrived at my office, marking him as a law enforcement agent of some sort. It began to make sense. This man had a clear understanding of my strategy from a different perspective, one as a law enforcement officer.

While I was still in my speechless phase, he continued. "It's all about networks, right? You know that Fred is the epicenter, and you obviously want to eliminate Fred. The problem is that Fred is volatile; too volatile to address directly. But Fred knows a guy named Frank and they have a relationship. Connect with Frank and you have a line to Fred. Another guy, Jack, knows both Frank and Fred. Marty does not know Fred, but he knows Frank and Jack really well. Affect any one of them and you affect Fred. It may be circuitous, but it is effective. In the end, it is all about Fred. Counterinsurgency strategy, right?"

I could do nothing but smile and nod my head in approval. In a few minutes, I readdressed the L4 attachment of the quadratus lumborum, finding it significantly less tender and less hyper-responsive to passive motion. Mr. K then stood up and tried gentle side-bending to the left, finding it to be quite comfortable.

"Fred is dead," he quipped.

HMOS, CEOS, AND HEADACHES

Mr. M came to the office complaining of relentless headaches that had been occurring for over three months. Since he was the head of an HMO, he had already been seen by various physicians and physical therapists. It was pretty clear there was no underlying pathology, something that is always a concern with headaches. He had underlying pathology amply addressed by the many medical resources at his disposal; now he was left with a clean bill of health and daily headaches! Various prescribed medicines did not seem to help him very much, and he did not like the side effects from them.

Mr. M had had headaches on and off in the past. These recent headaches were similar in intensity but much higher in frequency. (This is very important. Headaches that are a new occurrence, or radically different from previous headaches, should be checked out medically.) The four components of headache quantification are frequency, intensity, location, and duration. The fact that he was having headaches for multiple days makes migraine type headaches highly unlikely, as does the fact that the intensity was moderate to low, whereas migraine tends to be on the higher end of intensity.

As to location, Mr. M said that he feels them starting at the base of his neck and then coming straight up over the head just above his eye. He feels this bilaterally. (This is also one of the signs pointing to tension type headaches vs. other head-ache types.) Most interesting was the headaches worsened with long hours at his desk. Lest we immediately think stress from work, the headaches happen even when he is at home and not doing work related activities. If he spent any time at his computer, even on something fun, he ended up with a headache.

This verbal clue plus the visual inspection of his body posture was telling. It wasn't what he was doing at the desk; it was just being at his desk that initiated the headaches. Having them come on later in the day (other people had ruled out things like blood sugar fluctuations) mean that the cumulative effect of gravity was a problem. A glance at his postural presentation revealed a rather remarkable forward head posture.

When I remarked to him about a possible connection of the headaches to his posture, I could tell from his response that he did not exactly embrace the idea! Tough sell I thought, but fair enough. I decided to take a huge risk, one that could seal the deal or send him out the door for good. Cradling under his occiput, I lifted his head gently to show him how ideal alignment feels. I even pressed down on his head, accentuating gravity substantially. This overpressure had no negative effect at all; his body easily absorbed the additional stress. I then moved his head forward of the plane of gravity, accentuating his forward head substantially. I slowly and carefully accentuated gravity with his head in this forward position. As I described the physics of the alignment of the cervical spine and how changing the gravitation line redirects force, I steadily kept the moderate pressure on his neck.

As my explanation continued, (it might have been a bit longer than necessary) he began to look uncomfortable. When I asked what he was experiencing, he was astonished that this forward position of his head had replicated his daily headache, which he did not have five minutes ago. He then revealed his skepticism of the connection between headaches and alignment (as if I didn't already know this!) Being able to replicate his problem with simple position certainly clarified the relationship. There was nothing to say; no client education was necessary. Prior to this little test, extolling the benefits of aligning his structure correctly would have gotten nowhere since he did not connect his structure to the symptom. He experienced the relationship between posture and pain quite dramatically and in no uncertain terms.

The strategy of recreating discomfort by movement or position is called provocative testing. Since the point is to provoke symptoms, one does not do provocative testing without careful thought as to the risks and rewards of such a strategy. When done correctly, the relationship or condition is clearly defined. As a result, however, symptoms are provoked, and they do not always disappear immediately after the test. The practitioner must decide if provoking symptoms is a risk worth taking.

Over the next three sessions, Mr. M. and I slowly and methodically worked to lengthen the muscles in his neck that produced the forward head position which are also known headache influences. Most of the effort went into both the sternocleidomastoid muscle and the rectus capitis posterior minor. Both of these muscles are heavily involved in both headaches and forward head posture. At my urging, he also had one of his ergonomic staff alter his workstation and he took more frequent breaks during the day. I'm happy to report that he now rarely has a headache, and he has a newfound respect for thoughtful hands-on approaches to the treatment of pain.

You can tell whether a man is clever by his answers. You can tell whether a man is wise by his questions.

- Naguib Mahfouz

THE RIGHT QUESTION

"Wow, this is fantastic! These techniques will be so helpful for one of my clients. I have never treated the hamstring in this position."

I always like to hear statements like this at one of my seminars; it assures me the material has immediate application by the participant. (So far, so good.)

"Do you have a client with hamstring issues?" I asked.

"Yes, well, sort of. My client is a star high school football player mostly because he is the fastest kid on the field. He plays offense, defense, and returns kickoffs. His mom is a client of mine and asked me to do sports massage for him just for maintenance. I discovered he has very tight hamstrings, even though they do not bother him. I have been aggressively treating his hamstrings for weeks with no real gains. His mom and I have been after him to stretch before practice and before games, but he doesn't really like that. We are trying to convince him that if he stretches out his hamstrings, he will be even faster and less likely to be injured. He doesn't seem convinced. In fact, he has become a bit negative towards treatment and doing his stretching. He feels as though he is now a step slower, which his mom and I think is the tightness finally catching up to him. These new approaches should help. Do you have any additional advice?"

"Yes. Stop what you are doing."

The therapist looked at me quizzically, wondering what that statement meant.

"Seriously, I'd suggest that you stop aggressively treating his hamstrings with the intent of lengthening them. I'd also suggest that you not make him do static stretches before practice or before a game. What you are doing could be very counter-productive."

Many times over the years, certified athletic trainers and I have mused about the hamstring tightness we found in athletes who have tremendous speed. We wondered if these athletes could be better with a more normal hamstring length or, conversely, do their tight hamstrings contribute to the blazing speed that makes them so valuable? (One does not experiment with elite athletes who make megabucks, but it does make for interesting conversation.)

The answer to our theoretical question came in 2009, when researchers at Nebraska Wesleyan University explored the relationship of speed and hamstring length with NWU track team. The results (published in the January 2009 issue of the Journal of Strength and Conditioning Research) were quite surprising. In their findings, the fastest runners generally had the tightest hamstrings. More importantly, the runners with tight hamstrings had an extremely efficient gait as measured by the amount of oxygen used during a run. Runners with the most flexible hamstrings were slower and *less* efficient.

As to the stretching before competition or practice, the data again isn't very convincing. A study of 1400 runners by USA Track and Field found that runners who stretched (using typical static stretching) and runners who didn't stretch had exactly the same injury rate.

"I'm stunned," my student exclaimed. "This is in conflict with what I have been taught."

"I understand. Nothing ruins a good theory like a few facts. Our profession, like so many others, often makes some major assumptions and teaches theory or philosophy as though it were fact. Our particular bias is that muscular tightness is the source of all pain. Think of it this way: How can a person in pain visit so many practitioners and get a different diagnosis from every one of them? If you see a neurologist, the diagnosis is neural in nature. If you see a physical therapist, lack of strength is the problem. A chiropractor will find the cause to be misalignment in your spine. If you see a massage therapist, the problem is due to muscular tightness. Each discipline has a bias, a lens through which the problem is seen. That bias is both our strength and an enormous blind spot. All of us need to be vigilant in questioning the assumptions we make based on that bias."

"I am really confused. Should I keep treating him? What should I do now?" she asked with hesitation.

"I'd continue to treat him, not with intent of aggressively lengthening his hamstrings, but to keep them functioning at maximal capacity. Trigger points in his hamstrings will reduce strength and more importantly, increase the possible onset of fatigue, which changes the firing pattern. Hamstring fatigue tends to increase as the season wears on, especially if he is playing so many minutes. You might plan on seeing him more as the season progresses. Keeping that hamstring healthy is the goal, not lengthening out to some idea of what is considered normal."

"I will do that. You know, I just realized something. Treatment protocols are like answers. Anyone who comes to see me with something specific is looking for an answer to their soft-tissue problem. I know how obvious this sounds, but before I can come up with the appropriate answer, I have to be absolutely sure it is in response to the right question. I think I have been focusing too much on the answer and not enough on the question. I can't believe I never thought of it like that before."

A wave of satisfaction passed though my body and I could only smile in response to her epiphany. Anything else she learned during that seminar paled in comparison to the magnitude of that lesson. Moments like that are the gems that make teaching so rewarding.

SECTION TWO:
FAILING AND LEARNING

Often during one of my seminars, I have participants stand up and notice subtleties about weight displacement and balance. If you pay close attention, you will notice the constant shifting of balance registered in your feet. The muscles of your legs and feet are constantly reacting (through proprioception) to the movement of your body during standing.

When you ponder that, it is quite remarkable. We often think of standing as a static, rather than dynamic, act. Politicians, being sure that they are correct, take a stand on an issue. Statistically, you are balanced only about two percent of the time during standing. The other ninety eight percent of the time you are correcting, otherwise known as falling. (If politicians understood this, the world might be a better place.)

I often reflect on this while teaching a seminar. I fear that students think that I have answers immediately available to whatever soft-tissue problem comes through my clinic door. Nothing could be farther from the truth. My life in the clinic is one of trying to understand the problem, intervening, correcting course, intervening, correcting, etc. I do this based on my knowledge gained through intense study plus many thousands of sessions over the years. While I may presently know more than I did years ago, I am also aware of countless other possible causes for the same symptom. The questions always increase in number faster than the answers.

It is with slight embarrassment that I look back to my earlier years. As a rather clueless but very sincere therapist, I discovered neuromuscular therapy (NMT) and jumped in whole heartedly. What I shudder to remember is how quickly I went from cluelessness to bravado. I felt NMT was the missing link in health care and that it was the answer to all pain. Being filled with answers, I didn't spend much time with questions and certainly did not notice inconsistencies and inadequacies in my skill set, philosophy, or practice results.

There is a fascinating principle called the Dunning-Krueger effect that reflects my early years. In essence, the people who know the least are the most confident. The people with more knowledge are acutely aware that there might be important information that they do not know.

As a clinician and as a leader of organizations, I struggle with this principle every day. Leadership is often seen in the model of a George Patton, a very authoritarian and confident style. The research and writing of Professor Jim Collins (author of "Good to Great" and "How the Mighty Fall"), paints a very different picture. Many great leaders question themselves, get consensus, are good listeners, and correct constantly as they gather more accurate information. The often stated fear is that listening and struggling can be seen as weakness.

This perception of weakness is often feared by clinicians as well. My personal experience in the clinic is that very few people see my willingness to admit I do not know an immediate solution to their pain as weakness. Many have remarked that my honesty was the first time a health provider actually admitted not knowing. Most have had health providers bluntly prescribe a treatment protocol with complete confidence, only to dismiss them after it didn't work. To admit not knowing is not a dead end, it means that we work together to figure out an answer. It is messy and circuitous, but I know of no other way.

In short, there is no learning without failing. Being willing to fail, listen, and correct course is the hallmark of a good therapist (and much else in life).

Together we have learned where nettles grow;

Where not the vanquished but the living sup.

What Galahad, enchanted, did not know;

The Grail is in the seeking, not the cup.

Samuel Hoffenstein

LEARNING THROUGH THE STRUGGLE

Mr. C came to my office at the request of his doctor and his physical therapist, both of whom I admire greatly. He presented with pain in the mid-thoracic area, at about T8-9 on the right side only.

The pain started about four years ago after long hours of sitting over a microscope. At first episodic, it slowly increased in frequency and intensity. Mr. C stated that if he changes position, the pain lessens almost immediately. If he is recumbent or supine, the pain disappears. When he awakens, he has about 30 minutes with no pain. Gravity seems to be his enemy; as long as he is out of gravity, the pain is gone.

Before Mr. C got on my table, I had him stand and side-bend to the left, which created a pull on the right side. Right side-bending against resistance also elicited pain, but less so. Passive flexion to the right lessened the pain.

I remember clearly Mr. C responding to a perplexed look on my face when I finished taking him through these movements. He kindly asked if I had any idea what the problem was (my facial expression sure wasn't giving him any confidence!)

"This worries me," I confessed. "It seems way too obvious, way too easy. Every time a problem seems easy, it often turns out to be enormously complicated. Your doctor and physical therapist are two of the best I know. If this problem is as simple as it seems, they would have solved it by now. Everything points to a muscular cause. If you had an intrajoint issue as the source of your pain, side-bending you into the pain should have made it worse. Stretching and contracting the muscle elicits symptoms. Let's approach this in the simplest way first. I am going to carefully and thoroughly treat the muscles in the area where you feel the pain. We will know soon enough if that helps."

The next morning, he called me as instructed and reported there was marginal improvement; it took about 15 minutes longer after awakening before the pain set in. Two days later, I saw him again for a short session. His symptoms were essentially unchanged. The last two days were right back to 30 minutes pain-free upon awakening, followed by the rest of the day being uncomfortable.

I have now seen him several times; the results are completely underwhelming. I tried referring him back to his doctor and physical therapist, but they don't know what to do for him either. I sent both of them a report of possible sources for his pain and the strategies I used to address each of these possibilities. The summary letter was essentially this: Here is what Mr. C describes, here is what I thought it might be, and this is what I did to address the problem from that perspective. None of these strategies worked. What they sent me back was a very complimentary letter about my reasoning and differential assessment capabilities and sent Mr. C right back to me, wishing me the best of luck.

I could walk you through all the different strategies I did and why I thought each of them might be valid. However, I think there is a much more valuable lesson in this case, one that I don't see talked about very much.

I have taught continuing education seminars for many years. In those courses, it often helps to share an example where the application of some treatment made a profound difference in someone's pain. The purpose is meant to give value and meaning to the information, to show the potential impact of the technique being presented.

There is, however, a possible downside to these successful case stories, including the ones I share with you in my various writings. I often get the sense that students think that every client visit is like a CSI episode- each case is solved in an hour after insightful assessment and skillful treatment. Keep dreaming. In real clinical life, there are very few silver bullet treatments, where one session does it all. Mostly, people come to the office with musculoskeletal discomfort that could have several possible causes. Figuring out the ultimate source takes time. By the second, most often the third session, the source is clearer and results may soon follow.

The important lesson in the story of Mr. C is that the struggle is everything. If a client presents with something you solve easily, you have learned nothing. Clients like Mr. C are the real teachers for therapists like you and me. We cannot know everything and they don't expect us to. What they do expect is that we will search for new strategies, comb the literature, ask more experienced colleagues, or refer them elsewhere. The searching exposes us to strategies that may help other clients in the future, even if it does not help this particular client. In this way, our personal knowledgebase of possible causes for and particular symptom keeps growing, giving us more tools for future clients with the same presentation.

If you are that therapist who struggles, who sincerely wants to help the people who grace your door but the process takes longer than you'd like, welcome to the real world. Learning is messy, but process of learning is everything.

Addendum: After writing this story and publishing it in Massage and Bodywork Magazine, Mr. C did indeed improve. Here is the rest of the story.

In an additional contact with his PT, she happened to mention that Mr. C also had a suspected disc issue in his lower neck. Remembering the writings of Dr. Robert Maine and his emphasis on a possible connection between lower cervical neural issues and mid-thoracic pain, I added neural work to our treatment. Almost immediately, Mr. C had marked improvement. The difference was astounding. All the hard work in the world, done in the wrong place, will not bring results. I believe this strategy was the thirteenth one I tried, but it was a winner. You may find it amusing to know that I also saw someone with his exact presentation a few weeks later. Of course, I tried strategy #13 first and failed miserably. In her case, it was strategy #2. I am forever humbled by life in the clinic.

Success consists of going from failure to failure without loss of enthusiasm.

- Winston Churchill

SOMETIMES YOU'RE THE BUG

Sometimes the biggest lessons in therapy aren't as provider, but the receiver. As the song says: Sometimes you're the windshield, sometimes you're the bug.

In 1994, I went with a small group of people to provide services for the indigenous poor in the mountains of El Salvador. The area we served is called Morazon, a place ravaged by the civil war. The tragedies that these people endured are beyond my comprehension; almost everyone had lost a family member in some horrible way or another during the years of civil war.

For the rest of my small team, being there was an adventure they had looked forward to for many months. All of them had been to El Salvador previously. For me, I was overwhelmed at the poverty I saw. I was not prepared for how visceral that image of poverty was; I felt like someone had punched me in the gut when watching very hungry and dirty children looking at me curiously. Since getting to this place was so difficult, we brought nothing in for ourselves, only a change of clothes. The rest of our luggage space was filled with supplies for the people of Morazon. We ate what they gave us; the women seemed honored to prepare and share what little food they had. When our team walked away from the dinner table leaving about half what was served, the children could be heard descending on the food as we departed. It made eating difficult; what we ate was taken from someone's share.

The idea for my participation in this trip came from a conversation I had with a physician friend of mine who had gone the year previously. He told me how rewarding the trip was, but that it was also very frustrating. There are three main health problems, parasites, respiratory issues, and musculoskeletal pain. The parasites are contracted from drinking contaminated water. Doctors can give them medicines to eliminate the parasites, but people will immediately be reinfected at the next drink of bad water. Fixing the water problem is massively complex and expensive, far beyond the current capabilities of solving. The people cook in their adobe homes where there are no chimneys. The house is completely filled with smoke during food preparation; the intense smoke is the source of their respiratory issues. The people believe that the smoke also kills any insects in the grain that they also store inside the house. This may be true but if the smoke is strong enough to kill bugs, it isn't great for human lungs either. The doctor also lamented at how best to treat muscular pain. Whatever medicine he had to treat pain would be gone in a couple weeks, leaving the people to suffer again. I commented that teaching the people how to treat each other using manual therapy could possibly provide relief at no cost and would not be dependent on the generosity of the outside world. (As soon as I finished saying that, I realized I had just volunteered!)

There were several lessons I learned in this trip to Morazon, all of them have stuck with me.

First, as we arrived in San Salvador and prepared for the trip into the mountains, I felt very uneasy. This uneasiness began during the flight to El Slavador. The goal of the trip was very simple; I would teach community members simple neuromuscular techniques so that these community health promoters could treat people in pain. What scared me was whether this endeavor was a better idea than a reality. Would this really work? Could I teach people effective techniques in a few hours? Would they be receptive? What if this was ill-conceived from the beginning? These people are depending on me and I have no assurance that this mission will be successful.

On our way in, we stopped to have lunch with a Salvadoran doctor who ran a small clinic. This clinic was not as remote as where we were going, but on the way. Our lunch was interrupted by a patient who came to the clinic for help with a headache. The doctor excused herself from the lunch, but I could not resist going back to see how she was treating this woman. The doctor's assistant took me back to the "pharmacy" where the doctor was looking for something to give the patient for her pain. The "pharmacy" was a cabinet with about five bottles of medicine, most of them over-the counter cold medicines, aspirin, and Tylenol. I was stunned.

I asked the doctor if it was appropriate for me to treat the patient; the relief on the doctor's face was visible. The woman's headache (luckily) seemed to be cervicogenic in nature, thirty minutes later she was quite a bit better. However much better the woman felt, I felt better still. I knew in my heart that I really did have something of practical value to offer these people. I ended up seeing three more people with that doctor, each of whom had muscular pain which I treated successfully. I left feeling elated.

During the following days, I would teach selected community members called health promoters how to perform simple manual treatments for muscles of the back and neck. Health promoters are community volunteers who learn rudimentary health care to be shared with the community. In the afternoon, I would treat people from that community who had muscular discomfort and pain. This served both as a clinic for the community members and also an opportunity to demonstrate these techniques to the health promoters I trained that morning.

The second day I was in the communities of Morazon, I was humbled by a lesson in how pervasive the belief that medicine alone can provide relief and healing really is. At lunch, I happened to glance up in the mountains and saw a tiny figure in a clearing. When I pointed this out to my translator, she told me this figure in the distance was probably a man coming to see me, a two hour walk from the clearing where he was presently. (Wow- I can't get people to come to my office if they have to park more than 50 feet away). Sure enough, later that afternoon this older man appeared. I greeted him with a smile and the translator relayed this man's description of his pain to me. His problem sounded like something I could help, but the man asked if we had medicine for his pain. The translator replied that we did not give medicine, but that I treated only with my hands. The man smiled, thanked us, and turned away to walk back home.

I was stunned, absolutely stunned. Here is a man in one of the most remote areas of the planet who believes that only a pill can help his pain. (To give you an idea about how remote this is, I had gone to great trouble to create a little manual in Spanish. It might as well been Swedish; none of these people could read and had very little previous access to books.) How inculcated can the belief in the power of pills be if an old man in this remote area would walk more than two hours for help and then turn around because we did not dispense medicine?

My second lesson was a very personal one which began the day we were to leave the mountains. Unfortunately, I unknowingly drank untreated water the evening before. I awoke to what I thought was thunder in the distance until I realized that the sound was coming from my intestines. "Lightning" soon followed the "thunder". Boy, did it ever "rain". I spent the morning in the latrine, it wasn't fun, plus, I felt terrible and very weak. The hike out of the mountains was absolutely one of the hardest physical trials I have ever endured. It would have been mildly difficult anyway, but being sick made it just awful. After hours of hiking and carrying our packs, we met our driver who drove us down from the mountains. I rode in the back of the Jeep, lying on top of the packs, getting bounced airborne for hours while we descended on what they called "roads".

After leaving the mountains, I noticed a new symptom. Every breath I took was accompanied by sharp pain on my left side, from my upper back down my left arm. Only if I breathed extremely shallowly would it not stab me. Not only had I defecated everything but my shoes, now I was sure that I had suffered a heart attack. By the time my flight from San Salvador arrived in Champaign, I looked like death warmed over. My wife took one look at me and marched my ailing body right to the ER.

For better or worse, the doctor was a client at my office and someone I admire. (I couldn't decide whether this was good or bad...) He is a brilliant man and an osteopath by training. I now shudder with embarrassment at how I detailed (okay, maybe blathered on) about my possible heart attack. Mildly ignoring my blathering, he asked me to inhale and bam, there was the knife in my left upper back and down the arm. He then asked me to turn my torso to the left and inhale and bam, there it was again. He then asked me to turn to the right and inhale; miraculously, my heart got better on the spot. Let's see, turn to the left and the pain is there, turn to the right and the pain is gone. Hmmm. Cardiac issue? I don't think so... How did I not notice this before?

It took me a few seconds to process this information. Mechanical pain (pain that is made better or worse with movement or position) is the domain of my profession! I teach this stuff! When the reality of the movement and pain relationship sunk in, my gaze met his. Before he could say anything, I thought I'd deprive him of stating the obvious.

"We are never going to have this conversation, okay?"

He just smiled. I thought I might get away without him saying anything in retort, but the temptation was just too great for him.

"Would you like me to write a script for you to see you?"

I didn't even answer him as I got up to leave. One embarrassed smile was all he got. As we exited the building and started to the car, my wife (who was in with me the whole time) looked at me and said, "What just happened in there?"

"Sometimes you're the bug," I murmured while strapping on the seat belt.

She looked at me, thought about asking for clarification and decided it just wasn't worth it. It was a pretty quiet ride home for a guy who had miraculously recovered from a heart attack.

ELATION AND DISAPPOINTMENT

Ms. L sat on the edge of the treatment table, looking at me with eyes that clearly reflected her pain and trepidation. She shifted her position frequently, a sign of nervousness more than pain, as she waited for some confirmation and clarification. Seth Will, one of my teaching staff, and a few of my students taking an advanced training were with me. In this particular training, we invite people who have pain in the area we have been studying to come for treatment. These clients know that they will be treated in front of the group, with one therapist taking the lead. Sometimes, it is one of the students in the class who treats the person (Some serious pressure: doing a treatment in front of your peers and teacher and then having to explain later about the decisions you made and why you made them). Since Ms. L was one of the first clients, the plan was for me to take the pretreatment history and Seth to take the lead role in treatment.

After giving me a few details, Ms. L asked a very fair question. "Why do I hurt so much? What is wrong with me? I am sure this is due to the accident, but I don't know why the pain is so bad. It did not start right away, but now it is terrible."

Ms. L went on to describe her whiplash in detail. After her history, I measured the range of motion of her neck. Extension and flexion were extremely limited, as was rotation to either direction. Hearing the extent of her limitation only confirmed to Ms. L that something indeed was terribly wrong with her neck.

Seth began with a very careful palpatory assessment of her tissue. He found exquisite sensitivity in several muscles that affect both rotation and extension. Ms. L was astonished at how location precise these tender areas were. One spot could be incredibly tender and yet a centimeter away would feel quite normal. Seth patiently explained the role of each muscle he addressed and how it played a role in both her restriction of range and possibly her pain. More than once, she acknowledged trigger points that perfectly replicated the symptoms she had been experiencing. Seth slowly released these points and kept returning to sensitive areas looking for a decrease in restriction and pain.

At the end of the session, Seth had Ms. L sit up to recheck her cervical range again. He had done that numerous times while she was supine to check his progress, but this time we finished by having her sit up in exactly the same way we started the session. As she sat up, I began to remeasure her extension as I had done earlier. Instead of 25 degrees, I stopped her from going any father when she edged past 60 degrees, only because I chickened out, not because she felt she should stop. The change was astounding! Before I could ask, she immediately checked cervical flexion (which was similarly improved) and then immediately into right and left rotation.

"Oh my God!" she exclaimed and then repeated twice (in a voice so loud it startled us). "I can't believe this! What did you do?" (For a second, Seth looked like he had just been accused of something. . .)

It was at that point that the tears came rolling down her cheeks. I have seen this many times in my career, but it always astounds me. The elation of improvement is often followed by the realization that years of needless suffering have occurred. Here was a woman who realized that she had been in pain for two years, thinking it was perhaps a permanent injury of a serious nature and an hour of muscular treatment had changed it. While initially thrilled, the realization that there was an answer all along was too much for her to bear.

"How could that be? What did you do? Surely, just massage and muscles could not do that."

That is one of those questions where it is a bit hard to know how to reply. I looked at Seth, he looked at me, and we both decided to let the irony of the question hang in the air.

As we explained what role each muscle played in her movement and pain limitations, I got the sense that Ms. L wasn't exactly paying attention. She just kept turning her head from side to side, waiting for the moment when the improvement would vanish as quickly (and in her mind, just as mysteriously) as it came. She repeatedly asked the same question; "Could muscles alone be the cause of such pain?"

As I walked her out of my office, she tearfully thanked me, while at the same time expressing astonishment. It was a rollercoaster of emotions going from the initial fear that something was permanently wrong, to elation in the improvement, to fear that the improvement would not last, to disbelief that non-invasive soft-tissue treatment could do what other treatments had not done. Her sincerity of emotions encapsulated that which I have seen many times before, but most people do not express the full range of these emotions so vividly.

You may think the story ends here, but, alas, it does not. I received an email from Ms. L about two weeks after our session. She had returned to her native Brazil and had an appointment with a doctor to see what was "really" wrong with her neck. The range of motion improvement we accomplished had largely stayed, but she still had some pain in original area of her neck. She was hoping the MRI could get to the bottom of this pain, which <u>had</u> to be more than just muscular.

I was stunned and disappointed. In one hour her range of motion and her pain had improved more than in two years. Instead of seeing this improvement as an opening for further progress, she ultimately dismissed it because of a belief that muscles alone could not cause so much pain and that muscular treatment could not create such improvement. Even the power of her personal experience was overridden by her belief system about lowly muscles and simple hands-on treatment. If dramatic improvement doesn't inspire confidence, what will?

SHOOTING THE GENERAL

First, a confession. I absolutely love skeptical clients. There is something enormously gratifying to me when a new client has serious doubts about the value of soft tissue therapy. Perhaps it stems from the fact that respect for my profession is not given, it is earned. I take great pleasure in earning respect by clearly and rationally stating what I think is wrong, what I am going to do, and the scientific underpinnings of the process undertaken.

Mr. Z was not skeptical, however, he was rude. There is a severe difference. He wasn't just doubtful about the efficacy of soft tissue therapy; he thought this was a waste of time. I think I know what you are thinking; how in the world did he end up in the office in the first place?

I saw Mr. Z at the request of his wife, who I have never met but is a friend of a friend. I agreed to see him to evaluate whether or not I could help him (When I am not sure whether I can help, I seldom charge people for the time.) My schedule is packed for weeks in advance, so the only option was for me to see him on my day off. Somehow, and I don't know how, his wife convinced him to come to my office. Once there, he was very clear about his feelings about the prospects of success.

"I have a serious problem, so serious that I have not been able to work for years" he stated. "No one seems to be able to help me, except for the meds that they give me. They don't help a lot, but at least it is something to help manage the pain."

"I have read the physician's report from both the surgeries. I have seen the X Ray and MRI reports. You had major surgery and your doctors are some of the best surgeons I know. What was done was necessary and appropriate, but unfortunately I understand you still have pain."

"Maybe they just didn't fix it correctly, because I still hurt."

"That is a possibility, but really a remote one. If the accident caused enough trauma to necessitate that kind of repair to your spine, think about the damage and trauma to the muscles and soft tissue in your back."

"Yeah, but this pain couldn't be muscular. It hurts too much and the muscular stuff should have healed years ago. Besides, you rubbing on it for a little bit is only going to be temporary help at best. I can't see how this will solve anything. I don't need to be pampered, I need real help."

At this point, I could feel my heart rate speed up and my stomach tighten.

This wasn't just doubt, it was dismissal and disrespect.

"First, the idea that muscular pain hurts less than pain of other origins doesn't hold water. A muscle spasm can bring you to your knees in a hurry. A muscle spasm in the back is rated second to the pain from a kidney stone on the severity scale. Second, good therapy can make lasting changes, something I have seen thousands of times in my thirty some years of practice.

"OK, maybe muscles are the cause of pain for many people, but I still believe that mine is caused by the original trauma and maybe not the best of medical care. If the original injury could be fixed, I think my pain would be gone."

"Let me explain something. The force it takes to create the kind of injury you suffered is off the charts, enough to fracture some amazingly strong structures. Surrounding this tough framework are nerves, muscles, and tendons that also suffered tremendous trauma. What is worse, those structures probably were further injured in the surgery which is unintended but true nevertheless. Research studies show that supportive muscles around the spine are injured and thus do not support your spine after surgery as they are supposed to. This can lead to further pain.

Mr. Z looks at me skeptically. "That may be true, but the real injury was to the spine itself. If that was just better, all the other stuff would disappear."

At this point, I laid down the main point of my defense.

"I get the feeling that you think if you shoot the general, the war is over. Unfortunately, we have many examples of the fallacy of that kind thinking. In reality, even though the initial trauma was to one structure, that kind of trauma also affected the surrounding tissue as well. Worse yet, some injured muscles are not doing the job they were intended to do, so other muscles have to make up the slack. Those muscles will soon lose their sense of humor about this new job description, so they too will start to complain.

Imagine it this way: a group of workers all assigned to complete a task. Normally, everyone works reasonably hard and no one is overburdened. There are certainly some workers that are more productive than others, but the system works. Suddenly, there is an unfortunate event and a few workers from the group are removed. The remaining workers have to do more; the same job must be accomplished with fewer workers. How does this happen?"

"Well, everybody has to step up to the plate and do more", asserted Mr. Z.

"That is a great idea, but is that your experience on any job site you have ever worked?"

Mr. Z looked down for a minute before shaking his head.

"Exactly, the workers who are already doing too much will try to do even more, because they see what needs to be done. The slackers will do even less because they see what is to be done as completely overwhelming."

Reluctantly, Mr. Z was nodding his head in agreement. He should know, having worked in construction all his working life. Under stress, those who do, do more. Those who have a tendency to underperform, under stress, do less. With regard to muscles, the same is true.

"I'd bet that the soft tissue is quite possibly the source of some of your pain for three reasons: the original trauma, the surgery itself, and the compensation that resulted. I cannot tell you that this work will solve your pain, nor can anyone else for that matter. The surgeons who did the repair could not tell you that, but they did the surgery based on a reasonable judgment of the possible outcomes. In this case, the question is whether or not soft tissue may play some role in your pain and the evidence seems to say that it is indeed possible. How much treatment of your soft-tissue will affect your pain is unclear. There is every reason to believe that soft tissue may account from 30-70% of the daily pain you feel. Could be more, could be less. There isn't really a down side to this, except for your time. I need to be careful about stirring up the waters by over-treating, but that is about the only negative. As to cost, I am willing to see you for a few times at no financial risk to you. If it helps, you pay me. If not, you owe me nothing. Game?"

At this point, Mr. Z agreed to allow me to examine the musculature of his back. I expected to find some sensitivity but I found much more than I had expected. Mr. Z was also surprised at the amount of sensitivity I was finding in his back and he was clearly getting into the idea that soft-tissue may play a role in his pain. With each place I found, he encouraged me to go after the restriction, as though it were an enemy to be conquered. Happy that I had shown him how sensitive and specific muscle problems can be, I was all too willing to do more work, both in intensity and duration that I would have otherwise.

I should have known better. When I called Mr. Z two days later to see how he was doing, he was not very happy. His pain had escalated since leaving my office. While he initially felt better after leaving my office, that night was terrible. The next day wasn't good; he had much more pain than he normally felt. This was just beginning to abate at the time I called. Needless to say, he wasn't thrilled with the idea of a repeat performance. While this is understandable, the situation is now a bit different than just two days ago. I needed to see him again, and soon.

"I understand your reluctance at coming in to my office for another treatment, but I just want to point out a couple of things. First, the major question we faced initially is whether or not soft-tissue could be involved in your pain. The answer to that is most assuredly yes, as evidenced by your reaction. If muscles had nothing to do with your pain, then treatment to them would have no positive effect, but no negative effect either. That the muscles responded so vehemently to the treatment is proof that they are indeed involved, especially since the resulting pain is exactly the pain you always have, only worse. We may have stepped on the dragon's tail, but at least we know where the dragon lives. To do nothing further is not going to solve the problem. The dragon will quiet down over time, but he has a long-term lease unless we address it. Now that I know the context, the approach will be very different. I'd like you to come in for two or three short sessions, about twenty minutes or so in length and all three within the next two weeks. I won't charge you, but we need to do this."

Reluctantly, Mr. Z agreed to come back in to the office. During the session, he quickly got over his fear of being treated and soon wanted me to be more aggressive. This time, I knew better. He left the second session feeling as though I could have done more to help him. Symptoms were quite a bit better after the next session, and he came into the third session a different guy. Instead of being dark and rather bitter, he had a smile on his face as he reviewed his present condition. He admitted that he was clearly better, as evidenced by his activity level. He was doing work around the house that he had not done in years and this clearly both pleased and surprised him. As he reported his improvement, I stayed as unemotional as possible (we Norwegians are quite good at that). I wanted him to acknowledge the improvement and make a commitment to getting better. At this point, I had not charged him for any sessions.

I wish I could end the story by saying that Mr. Z came for subsequent sessions, improved greatly, and began to resume his previous activities. Instead, he told me over the phone that since my work was not covered by insurance; he did not want to continue. If money was at the heart of the issue, I would have done everything possible to see him. From what I know about his situation, money was not the issue. In reality, I have no idea why he elected not to pursue treatment. For whatever reason, he chose not to pursue something that he admitted had helped him more than anything else. When he stated his intention not to return for more sessions, I did not react at all except to acknowledge his decision.

Upon hanging up the phone, I walked down the hallway of my office to the door of my treatment room and knocked lightly on the door. A voice from inside the room said "Ready", and I began a new journey with another new client. Before walking into the room, I glanced up at the Japanese scroll hanging just outside my office door: "Every opportunity for service is an opportunity never again to return." Shaking off the past, I vowed to do my absolute best for the person inside my treatment room. She deserved nothing less.

YOU ARE GOING TO USE YOUR HANDS?

Today, in the midst of a really busy day, came a phone call that jolted me back to reality. Seeing one person after the other, surrounded by other therapists in my office doing the same thing, can be a very insular environment. It is easy to forget the rest of the world isn't on the same page.

I could see that my office manager was busy with three things at once so when the second line rang I picked up the phone, just before I went in session. I assumed this would be a quick phone call, with someone making or changing an appointment.

"You guys deal with people in pain, right?" (That was quite an opening line!) "I have a pain in my hip and I am wondering if you can help."

I patiently explained to the young man on the phone, I would guess him to be in his twenties, that this is exactly what we do. He described going to the emergency room a week ago and receiving a diagnosis of bursitis of the hip. He was not in an accident; it just came on over a two to three day period.

"They told me to make an appointment with an orthopedist as soon as I could. I called today to check on the time of my appointment and was told that the cost would be $480 for the office visit. The shot of cortisone, which the ER doctor recommended, would be an additional charge. I do not have health insurance and there is no way I can afford this. I am looking for an alternative."

"I understand your predicament. It is possible that the cortisone might be the only way to help your hip pain, but that is not absolute by any means. First, a simple strategy would be to address the soft tissue, the muscles and ligaments around your hip. If it is bursitis, tightness in a couple muscles around the hip could irritate the bursa, treating these muscles may reduce your pain. Second, there are muscles that perfectly mimic bursitis pain. If this is really your problem, it is possible that treating one of these muscles could make a big difference. In the worst case, soft-tissue has very little to do with your pain, and you are only out the time it takes to treat you and $50."

"OK, that sounds really good. That I can do. But how much would you charge for the shot?"

I explained to him that there would not be a charge, as we do not do injections.

"How much for the prescriptions though? I just need to know how much money this is going to cost."

Again, I explained that we don't use injections or drugs, just Precision Neuromuscular Therapy. The treatment is completely hands-on. There are no pills and no injections.

"Wait; you are just going to use your hands? What good would that do? (At this point, I was stunned!) Can you guarantee me that this will help? It sure doesn't seem like it."

"Before I further explain what I would do, may I ask you a question? Did the doctor's office guarantee that the cortisone shot would fix the problem? No? Call them and ask for a guarantee and see what happens. Here is what I am willing to do. Come to the office and let me take a look at your hip for 10-15 minutes. In that time, I should have a pretty good idea if this could help you. If the answer is no, then you leave without paying a dime. If it seems reasonable, then we will continue for no more than thirty minutes. You would probably need two treatments to make progress. If it doesn't help after two sessions, I will refund your money. You cannot lose."

"But there are no shots and no pills? Nothing? Can I talk to my girlfriend and call you back in fifteen minutes?"

As I hung up the phone, I knew darn well this kid was not calling back. In his mind, no shots, no pills, no way. This is not good for the physician either. Patients expect to walk in the door, get a shot and have a miraculous healing. Very seldom does treatment work so miraculously, for the orthopedist or for practitioners like me. Somewhere last night, there was a young man who was hurting and did not sleep well. Neither did I.

SECTION THREE: DIFFERENTIAL ASSESSMENT

One of the most important skills that can be developed in any therapist is the decision making process; to plot out the possible causes for any presenting symptom and methodically confirm or disconfirm each of them. This takes a skill set developed both by the acquisition of knowledge through study and the rich set of data from one's experience in the clinic.

When teaching, I often find that students would like to have a comprehensive protocol, a specific set of tests that would be applied to any symptom. Unfortunately, this would be a one-size-fits-nobody adventure and very time inefficient. While there are simple rules in the beginning, the flow chart can go in many possible directions for every possible symptom. While a bit daunting to learn, in the end, this is the most honest way I know to convey good clinical reasoning.

The real voyage of discovery consists not of seeking new land-scapes but in seeing through new eyes.

Marcel Proust

NOTHING IS AS IT SEEMS

At the urging of his wife, R came to my office to be assessed for his shoulder pain. He was a very personable man, but his skepticism was very apparent. I love seeing people who have that much doubt when they walk in my office. Every morsel of respect I get is something I have to earn, not something given to me by title or position. If the work and my skills are worthy, respect is a natural by-product.

R's pain was in the lateral aspect of the deltoid, right at the greater tubercle. When my staff and I (three of my staff were also present for the evaluation) inquired about the genesis of his pain, he reported that it started about sixteen months ago with a serious strain when lifting something. He had his arms overhead and tried to pull something forward; immediately he felt a searing pain in his shoulder. The pain mysteriously disappeared for many months, only to resurface in the last few weeks.

He had seen his doctor, who asserted that R probably had a bit of a tear in the rotator muscles, which had probably healed since the original injury. I agreed with his doctor. He probably did have some microtearing, which could not have been too serious since he had no pain or obvious loss of function for months.

Given the location of his pain and the fact that this happened while his arms were overhead, all signs pointed directly to the supraspinatus. I did resistive testing of the deltoid in multiple positions, none of which was weak or painful. When I tested the supraspinatus directly, it was very weak. Thinking this was going to be a very straight-ahead case, I quizzed my staff members about what our options were. All of us were sure this was the supraspinatus muscle, pure and simple.

I remember hearing that Henry Ford used to refuse any recommendation by a committee that voted with a unanimous vote. He believed that if everyone agreed, someone was not looking at all sides of the situation. There is always a shadow side, another possibility. Unanimous votes are like mob actions, people are not thinking for themselves. (Such wisdom from the guy, me, who was actually leading the mob.)

At any rate, when I had R lie on the table and examined the supraspinatus muscle, I could not find any area of restriction or sensitivity. The tissue felt totally unremarkable, both to me and to him. This was a total surprise. I was dumbfounded and was tempted to reexamine tissue I had already reexamined twice.

Resisting that temptation, I did have him sit up again while I retested the strength of his supraspinatus. It was still quite weak, only the tiniest bit better.

While I was resistive testing the supraspinatus, one of my staff noticed how much R was splinting with his upper trapezius. I was too focused on the supraspinatus to notice the shoulder hike. Aha, this is where the problem is...

For a guy who was as muscular as R was, I don't think I have ever felt such a healthy trapezius. I was stunned at how compliant and pliable the tissue was. I have more than a hundred clients who would love to have upper trapezius muscles that healthy. So much for the splinting idea.

This was getting seriously perplexing. Why does the supraspinatus test weak yet seem neither restricted nor sensitive?

I asked R if he could lie on his right side, to which he rather emphatically said "No". I asked "Why not" and he said that pain in his shoulder kept him from doing that. This was something that did not make sense given what I found with his supraspinatus. What would cause the pain in the shoulder from lying on his side yet explain the pain in the lateral aspect?

I asked R if there were any other motions that bothered him. He took his arm out to the side and did an external rotation with his humerus.

"This hurts. I can only get it to about right here before there is pain."

We quickly measured his external rotation capability. It was at 53 degrees; quite limited from the normal range of 90 degrees.

There are (at least) two possible reasons for this limitation: weakness in the external rotation muscles or tightness in the muscles that do internal rotation. Since he had pain while doing external rotation, it implicates the muscles creating the action. The muscles that create external rotation are the infraspinatus and the teres minor. Suddenly, I remembered that R also did not want to lie on his right side, which is common with infraspinatus discomfort. When there is an injury or trigger point in the infraspinatus muscle, this reduces microcirculation. The additional pressure of lying on that side reduces already reduced circulation even more, producing pain. The picture was getting clearer!

As I examined the infraspinatus, R's eyes widened.

"Whoa, that's tender!" he asserted. This was remarkable given that he hadn't said a thing about any spot I had pressed upon earlier.

"That is strange. When you press back there, I feel it down here," he said, pointing to his deltoid area. (Things were starting to look up!)

I carefully examined every millimeter of his infraspinatus, and there were some very tender areas, much of which recreated his symptoms. The test of the validity of this approach came in two forms: resistive testing of the deltoid and the ability to lie on the right side. Since he was already on the table, I asked him if he would mind turning on to his right side. He did and we waited for his report. R kept moving his arm, trying to get it in the exact position that bothered him at night, when lying on the right side for even a few minutes.

"There", he said, "I feel the pain when the arm is exactly in this position." He said this with the satisfaction of a kid who finally found a flaw, something which just seemed a bit amusing since the pain wasn't exactly subtle before I treated it.

"OK," I said. "Let's look at one more thing." I had him lie supine while I examined the teres muscles with a pincer palpation. As his eyes narrowed, I figured I must be on the right spot. As the tissue cleared, I had him roll back on the right side. He kept searching for a position that might recreate the pain, but it was taking him longer to find one.

At this point, I had R sit up, and I did resistive testing on the supraspinatus muscle. This time, the strength was significantly better, something that was obvious to me, to R, and to the therapists who were observing. Clearing the infraspinatus and the teres muscles of these trigger points had enabled these muscles to better stabilize the glenohumeral joint, something that is necessary for proper functioning of resistive abduction.

Addendum: The results of the treatment were really quite stellar. In one hour, he went from weakness and pain to strength and the ability to lie on his right side for the first time in recent memory. Like several other stories, this one did not have a fulfilling ending. The treatment I provided for him was free, but I told him that his responsibility in repayment was to call or email me in three or four days after our session. I needed to know whether or not the gains accomplished stayed. I also predicted it was likely that a couple more sessions were needed.

I did not hear from him, but I did see his wife about ten days later. She reported that his shoulder felt quite a bit better for several days, but then slowly reverted back to where it was previously. The first symptom to revert was his inability to lie on his right side. The pain and weakness returned in about one week. Even though his wife had encouraged him to return for a couple follow-up sessions, he declined to do so. His reasoning was that he is a busy guy and the work must have only provided temporary relief anyway. This is quite disheartening, but not altogether rare. It could mean several things, not the least of which is that I failed to convey to him that soft-tissue therapy a process, not an event. Or, he just decided that the process of resolving the pain isn't worth the effort. This is hard to understand but certainly his choice. Lastly, he may have had no faith the outcome would be favorable. If this were the case, his decision is hard to understand since he saw immediate improvement in just one session.

Whatever the reason, one learns to control only that which is under our own sphere of influence. I can do a better job of conveying the process of Precision Neuromuscular Therapy to clients from the beginning. The rest is up to the client.

MAN, THAT'S JUST WRONG

J was an athletic young man attending college on a basketball scholarship. Unfortunately, one day in practice, he had a terrific collision with a guy who should be playing football instead of basketball, and J suffered an immediate disc injury in his low back. At that time, he presented with all the typical symptoms of a low back and disc injury, which was a symphony in three parts; back pain, pain radiating to the buttock, and pain radiating down the leg. His athletic trainer and his doctor (both of whom are excellent) kept close tabs on him and helped him navigate through the injury process quite well. Using injections and other therapies, the inflammation of the disc seemed to be much reduced. In the usual course of events, the pain retreats to the original injury site, that is, the leg pain will abate first, followed by the pain in the gluteal area, and then finally the low back pain recedes.

Most perplexing to J and his medical team was the fact that while the disc showed clear evidence of healing, the pain in the legs remained. Even though the pain in the back and buttock was all but gone, the leg pain remained unchanged, if not worse. His trainer and doctor were perplexed; this is really an atypical progression for this type of injury. J was fearful that this could be a permanent condition that would impact his future in basketball.

I assessed J's structure and saw nothing of note that might be relevant to his pain. Having him lie supine on the treatment table, I assessed his hamstrings for length. His left hamstring was at 145 degrees, quite limited, but I have seen many hamstrings this restricted (the ideal length is 170 degrees). His right, the side of the pain, was at 115 degrees, which is probably the most restricted hamstring I have ever seen.

"Whoa. You weren't kidding about your hamstring being tight, this is really quite restricted. Tell me what happens when I stretch your hamstring. Is it painful or does it feel like the muscle just can't lengthen more than that? (If the stretch was painful, this could be a guarding response to protect the nerve rather than muscle tightness) Tell me where you feel it the most..."

"Right here" said J as he pointed to the bicep femoris belly.

Keeping the hamstring on a stretch, I asked J to arch his neck into extension and then bring his neck into flexion to see if that changed the sensation in his hamstring. No change. (If it did, the cause would be neural tension, not true hamstring shortness.)

"I think I can explain what is happening to your hamstring and how it relates to your original injury. Beyond the original trauma to the low back, which must have been pretty intense, the disc was clearly affected. Disc injuries often refer to the buttock, which probably explains why you felt pain there in addition to the low back. The disc injury often irritates a major nerve exiting the spine, either directly or by subsequent inflammation. The nerve is like a root system for a tree; as it travels downward it has many branches, one of which serves the hamstring and the muscles in the back of your leg. The progression is this; you injure the disc, which sensitizes the nerve. The nerve however, innervates all these leg muscles, which also become highly sensitized and therefore respond inappropriately to stimuli.

In the most logical progression, as the nerve heals, the muscles should too. The operative word here is *should*. Research has shown that muscles served by an irritated nerve root are more likely to develop something called trigger points than other healthy muscles. These trigger points can restrict range of motion, cause deep aching pain, or mimic the tingling or burning sensations of nerve irritation. Here is the irony; the trigger points in your leg replicate exactly the symptoms of the original injury, even though the nerve root inflammation has improved. Is that bizarre or what?"

J summarized the dilemma differently.

"So you are saying that the low back injury sensitized the disc, which caused the nerve problem, which then caused the muscles to hurt. Even though the low back and disc caused this mess, muscle pain, the third link in the chain, is now independent of the thing that caused it in the first place. It is like A causes B, B causes C, but C stays when A and B are better."

"That's pretty much the story," I replied as I nodded in agreement.

"Man, that's just wrong."

I'M SORRY, WAS I STARING?

"What a litany of practitioners you have visited", I remarked.

"Every one of them has a different diagnosis," she replied.

Ms. D came to my office with an interesting symptom presentation. She has suffered from intermittent back pain for two years, with occasional echoes of mild pain down the back of her leg. She has also had some occasional hip issues, nothing really long-lasting. The pain she has is more annoying than disabling. She can only walk for short periods of time before the pain worsens and causes her to sit down or lie down to relieve the symptoms. She was on a trip recently where she had to walk downhill frequently, which increased the pain markedly.

Ms. D began by outlining the number of practitioners that she has seen and what the various diagnoses have been. Her primary care doctor thought it to be some sort of disc issue, but did not do any follow-up studies or imaging. Anti-inflammatory drugs made only a marginal improvement. One physical therapist suggested an approach using prolonged passive spinal extension, which really made things worse.

When this did not help, she asked to see another physical therapist, who surmised that the problem was initially a hamstring issue (which is reasonable). An aggressive stretching routine was prescribed, which again made things worse, not better.

Seeing that this course was not working, she switched therapists. The new physical therapist concluded that the problem was an issue with the sacroiliac joint. Numerous manipulations were performed and Ms. D was given some exercises to do at home. Again, the results were underwhelming.

Somewhere in her description of her next foray with still another practitioner, this time a chiropractor, I found myself involuntarily drawn to glancing at her legs. Ms. D sat facing me, a rather pretty woman in a fairly short skirt; try as I may not to, I kept finding my eyes drifting to her legs. What was it that kept drawing me to her legs? I tried to pay attention to the description of her chiropractic experience, but I missed many of the details because my gaze kept returning to her legs. Something was noteworthy, but what? At some extremely embarrassing moment, she slowed down the speed of her talking, because she was aware of my gaze and I was aware that she was aware! I had just been busted (for a crime I didn't exactly commit-like actually scratching the side of your nose at a stoplight while the person in the other car thinks, well, you get the idea). For the life of me, I could not at that moment come up with a reasonable explanation for my actions. For a moment, the world froze. . .

"Excuse me," I said. "Was I staring"? (Brilliant observation Sherlock!)

At that moment, an epiphany happened and I knew what was bothering me about her legs (there is a God).

"I am sorry to be distracted, but I cannot help but be drawn to something. Have you noticed that your legs are not the same size?"

The look of surprise on her face said it all. I could tell she was internally weighing the idea that my statement was either a brilliant observation from an experienced therapist or a confirmation that I was really a nutcase. (I hadn't exactly instilled confidence in my professionalism at this point.)

"If you don't mind, may I take some measurements?"

We moved from the chairs to my treatment table where I had her lie supine. I retrieved a tape measure from my desk and wrapped it around the mid-thigh of her left leg. Being careful to measure at exactly the same place on the right leg, the difference in girth was six centimeters, a significant difference for someone of her size. She was stunned and sat up to look at her legs, comparing them visually. We could both see the obvious difference. I measured again and yet a third time. Each time, the numbers were the same.

She sat up, waiting for some light to be shed on the relevance of this discovery.

Reviewing all the different diagnoses that she had, what was the relevance of the leg girth differential? Would a hamstring issue cause this? Not likely. An SI joint problem? No. Piriformis issue? As we went through the possible reasons, the only one that made any sense was some sort of nerve root involvement that would create a slight atrophy on one leg.

"Wait," I said. "What did you say about your curve in your low back? I think I missed that earlier". (I missed it because I was otherwise occupied. . .)

Ms. D stated that her chiropractor had remarked that she was losing some of the curve in her low back. She had seen the chiropractor intermittently and this person noticed that the lordotic curve in her back was slowly decreasing. Even though she tried to counteract that by passive extension (called the McKenzie method, which is what one of the physical therapists had her do), it was just more comfortable to sit and stand in a flexed position. The extension, which was supposed to feel good if the problem was a disc issue, made the pain worse.

"I think you need to go back to your primary care doctor and request/demand an MRI. I think it likely that he was correct all along; it is a neural issue but not what he thought. Get the MRI."

Ms. D returned to my office for a chat in about five weeks. She had had the MRI, which showed exactly what I thought: stenosis in her lower spine. This explained her pain pattern and why she had been losing the curve in her low back. Flattening of the lumbar curve actually creates greater room in the foramen, something her body did instinctively to counteract the stenosis. Her doctor was surprised and impressed that a massage therapist weighed in with such important information.

For me, it was a very real lesson in what neuroscientists call "thin-slicing": the ability to extract, in an instant, multiple sets of data faster than the cognitive brain can process it (or explain it!)

THE CASE OF TROCHANTERIC BURSITIS, THAT WASN'T

KK is an energetic young woman with an infectious smile, only sixteen years old but amazingly mature for her age. She is a high level gymnast who has been struggling with pain in her hip over one year. She had been diagnosed with trochanteric bursitis and had visited various physicians and had a couple of rounds of physical therapy before coming to my office. Her condition did not improve, in fact, it worsened over time. Often, physicians would implore her to quit gymnastics for an extended time, which she finally consented to do. This did not help and she lost precious time in the search for an answer to her pain.

Seen as an intractable case of trochanteric bursitis, she was referred to a physician in Kansas City for removal of the bursa. (I didn't even know that was possible). Before the doctor would agree to remove the bursa, he wanted to confirm the diagnosis with one last test. He anesthetized the bursa and guess what? There was no change in her pain level. He informed KK and her parents that the bursa could not be the problem since anesthetizing had no effect on her pain. This was not good news since she had undergone nearly a year of treatment on the bursa. The doctor suggested that the family pursue the possibility that tightness in the soft tissue over the trochanteric head was causing the pain. (This was one very smart doctor!)

KK and her parents came to my office and we began treatment. Her pain was diffuse over the entire lateral flank, not a usual pain pattern for bursitis. The Ober test on the abductors showed moderate restriction, leading me to think that the doctor was right on the money. When the iliotibial band and the tensor fascia lata are very restricted, they have a tendency to cause friction over the trochanteric head every time the person goes from hip flexion to hip extension. Her hip was hypersensitive and the work had to be done extremely gently.

I saw KK about five times before the pain in the hip started to abate. KK and her parents were thrilled; this was the first relief she had in over a year. The Ober test showed marked improvement and the diffuse pain over the hip seemed much better. She began to think about resuming gymnastics and was very excited about the improvement. Finally, they had some hope that this condition could be resolved!

The progress however, revealed other distressing signs. While her hip pain was seemingly better, her ability to do gymnastics hit a serious wall. While walking was less painful, she felt a sharp stabbing pain every time she would load weight on her leg (on the involved side). This was very discouraging. All the soft-tissue influences around the hip were markedly improved. It seemed clear that the pain was coming from somewhere else. But where?

A common referral pattern from the quadratus lumborum is to the area near the hip. Following this lead, I examined her QL and found it to be very sensitive. Actually, a lot of the other soft-tissue around her back was also sensitive. When I remarked about how sensitive the back musculature was, she revealed that she had severely injured her back before the hip pain started. Additionally, the hip pain was immediately preceded by an unexplained groin pull or what seemed like a groin pull.

I thought this new information was indeed the crucial piece to the puzzle. With new-found hope, I carefully examined her low back musculature. While much of it was very tender, none of it referred directly to her hip. No single spot replicated her pain. This was not a good sign.

For reasons unknown to me at the time, I tried one other thing. If I gently pushed her L5 vertebra forward, she braced in pain and said that she could feel that go right to her hip. I could now replicate her hip pain perfectly with pressure and a precise stress to her low back. This became the new focus and I addressed multiple muscles and ligaments in her back. Any decrease in sensitivity gained during a session was lost within hours of her leaving my office. It was clear that the back was the issue and that what I was addressing was the effect, not the cause. Unfortunately, I had no other options to offer KK. This problem was something I neither understood, nor could help her overcome.

In desperation, I looked for other places to send her. I knew a local chiropractor I could send her to, and the family trusted my judgment. I went to the first appointment with them.

Oh boy, was that a learning experience! Mr. Slick DC came in to meet the mom and KK, greeting them with an air of confidence, bordering on cockiness. As he showed the x-rays to us, he explained his diagnosis and how he would have her back on the gymnastics mat in three weeks or less. He looked quite pleased with himself after his impressive display of confidence and clarity, which was soon to be shattered.

KK (remember she was sixteen) kindly, but firmly, reminded Mr. Slick DC that she had been to several specialists over the last year, many which had more impressive credentials than him and all of whom were just as sure of their diagnosis as he was. At this point, she stated that since they had been misguided and overconfident, she had no reason to believe he was any different. She would, however, do everything he asked and follow his instructions to the tee. If respect was in order, he would have to earn it. I'd like to share with you that Dr. Slick was looking quite disoriented at this moment, having been served a super-sized plate of the truth. I was sliding down in my chair, not knowing whether to snicker or bolt for the door.

KK followed the chiropractor's instructions to the tee. She came for treatment as often as he told her and did everything he asked her to do outside the clinic. Not unexpectedly, the results were nonexistent. No worse, no better. I must tell you that the family was a little miffed at me for making such a poor referral. That was an uncomfortable revelation for me and something I won't do again. I will never again refer a client to anyone in whom I do not have complete trust.

Looking at KK one more time, I reviewed in my head the possible reasons for her pain. What is it about the lower back that could refer pain to the hip? I had her replicate the pain for me in the office yet again. Almost every time she loaded weight on her leg with any kind of impact, the pain went right from her back to her hip. Wait, why wasn't it _every_ time she loaded her leg? What was the common factor for when the pain shot from the back to the hip? As I watched her gait and movements again, I saw it. Extension. Every time she loaded the leg with the least bit of extension, the pain was recreated. I figured it out! Wait; I still don't know what that means. I felt like a guy with the keys to a lockbox with millions of dollars in it, except I don't know where the lockbox is located.

Not knowing what to do, I told KK and her parents that I would do more research. Where I would find an answer I did not know, but I would keep trying. In the meantime, I asked them to continue looking for a specialist who could decipher the information I uncovered into something usable. The parents, an amazing and patient couple who doggedly pursued help for their daughter, finally found a specialist in Chicago who reviewed her CAT scans closely and found a stress fracture/pars defect at L5. He also took x-rays in multiple positions and saw the hot spot on the film. It had been there all along; the other doctors just did not see it (partially due to the fact that they did not look for it). After treatment from this specialist in Chicago, KK improved greatly and had just auditioned for college scouts, when we last talked.

This case was a big lesson for me; I really felt as if I had failed KK and her family. She had improved 50% under my care, but I could not help her to complete recovery. As it turned out, I could _not_ have helped her with her real problem. Being honest about my inability to help her caused the family to seek out the doctor in Chicago, who finally solved the problem. He told them that the best care and analysis she received during her painful ordeal was from the doctor in Kansas City and surprisingly, from a massage therapist in Champaign. Sometimes, the best way to help is acknowledging your ineffectiveness.

TOO YOUNG FOR A HEART ATTACK

When I walked out to the waiting room, C was sitting with his grandmother. He was in his early twenties but looked much younger, as he sat in the waiting room chair. Clearly in pain and/or worried, he looked like he was embarrassed and wanted to be anywhere else on the planet but in my office.

"Who sent you here?" I asked. "Tell me what has been going on."

C described how he had been traveling overseas and felt his neck begin to tighten. As much as he tried, he could not get it to stop. His range of motion was very limited, and he could not find a place where it would stop hurting. It seemed to spread into his upper trapezius area and upper back. Traveling in Europe didn't help and carrying luggage seemed to aggravate it.

After he returned to the States, he was alarmed to discover that he now had pain in the left side of his chest. This pain was faintly connected with breathing but not in the linear way that you would expect. This was obviously very disconcerting to him. His first thought was that he was having a heart attack, but he was only twenty two. How could that be?

Relaying his symptoms to his grandmother, she took him straight to the doctor's office. After some testing, it was clear that he did not have a cardiac problem. The source of his symptoms was diagnosed as musculoskeletal. The doctor sent him to my office, where they arrived without an appointment. Luckily, I had a cancellation and could see him immediately.

As C sat, I palpated his neck. His rotation had improved since the original onset of pain and was not substantially restricted; the movement just felt very stiff to him. The most restricted plane of motion I noticed seemed to be extension of the neck. His extension was moderately restricted, and I noticed there was a fair amount of muscular guarding while he was doing it.

Having him lie supine on my treatment table, I began to palpate his tissue. He had described very significant tightness in his mid-scapular area. I addressed his levator scapula, iliocostalis, and serratus posterior superior. All of this was tender to the touch, but nothing significant. No particular point replicated the pain he had been having in his upper back. Feeling no remarkable tissue abnormalities, I decided to go a different route.

Palpating the muscles of his chest, nothing stood out as significant. Again, everything I touched was somewhat sensitive, but nothing was "the pain".

At this point I could see that C was feeling good about having the areas worked but a little perplexed as to why I kept moving, not staying in any specific place to completely release the tissue.

"Have you ever heard of trigger points?" I asked. "Trigger points are like call forwarding for pain. Press in one place, and the person feels sensation somewhere else. It is an amazing phenomenon. Let me demonstrate."

At that point, I slowly began to search his left scalene muscles for tight bands of tissue. Within a minute, I found a tight band and nodule that was exquisitely tender.

"Holy crap!" he exclaimed. "That is crazy! I feel that right between my shoulders and into my chest. That is nuts! It is like you have your hand right into my back and into my chest at the same time. What the heck?"

At this point, I explained to C that this is exactly what a trigger point is. The reason that I could not locate the causative spot in his midscapular area or his chest is that there is no spot to locate. The sensitivity in his mid-back and chest are referred pain from the trigger point in his scalene muscle.

"I was so worried about the heart thing. Man, it felt like the big one or something."

"I would not worry about your heart. Check this out. I press here (pushing on his scalene), and you have chest pain, I let go of the spot and your chest improves immediately. I'd say that is a pretty clear relationship, wouldn't you?"

The relief and astonishment in his face was quite a sight; astonishment from the experience of the referral and relief in knowing that his heart was fine, and he would probably live through the week! His worried and submissive demeanor changed into that of a vibrant young man who has places to go and things to do. His grandmother shot me a look of gratitude as her grandson bounded out the door of my clinic. I am guessing they had quite an afternoon together.

HICCUPS

From the other room, I heard my office manager speaking with a woman on the phone.

Not surprisingly, the call came from the patient's wife. There was a back and forth movement to the conversation, I caught only a few morsels here and there. A little later, my office manager said that she had a case that was strange enough I might be really interested in tackling it.

"Ready for this? That was a woman on the phone who said that her husband has had hiccups for almost three weeks, and she is wondering if Precision Neuromuscular Therapy could help. I told her I wasn't sure, but that I would ask you to call her." (I think she left out the part about it being a strange case, and that I like strange cases. . .)

One does not think about such a simple action like a hiccup until it becomes pathology. Truthfully, what I knew about hiccups you could have put in a thimble. Since I had my office manager schedule the hiccup couple two days out, I had time to do my homework. A hiccup is basically a spasm of the diaphragm. While there are many short-term causes for hiccups (eating too fast, eating too much, drinking too much), there are also some very serious diseases that can cause hiccups (stroke, multiple sclerosis, tumors, etc.). I wasn't really worried about these possibilities though, as his doctor had eliminated any serious potential cause.

When the wife and her reluctant husband came into the office, both were at wits end. He was stressed because the hiccupping would not stop, and she because his hiccupping was driving her over the edge, as well. He was very frustrated, and I could tell that he thought this approach was doomed to failure, as the other interventions from his doctor had been.

There seemed to be two distinct approaches to affecting his hiccups: approaching the diaphragm directly or treating the nerve that serves the diaphragm, the phrenic nerve.

"When did this start?" I inquired. "Can you connect anything you did to the genesis of the hiccups?

Neither of them could think of anything directly related to the onset of the hiccups. All they could tell me was that the hiccups started about three weeks ago. He was in the hospital for a surgical procedure; it started after that.

"That just might be our cause," I said. "It is very possible that during the surgery there was some stress on the front of your neck, perhaps from a tube inserted in your throat. If there was some additional stress on the muscles in the front of your neck in the next day or so, that could be the cause."

"What does the neck have to do with hiccups?" asked the husband, looking more confused and lost than ever.

I got out one of my anatomy books and showed both of them the path of the phrenic nerve and its proximity to the scalene muscles. Given the local trauma from the surgery, his chronic forward head posture, and perhaps some post-surgical stress that he did not remember, it is reasonable to assume that the scalenes could be sensitizing the phrenic nerve by compression. It was at least a reasonable hypothesis.

I treated his anterior neck muscles very carefully, being careful not to intrude on the nerve, which would further traumatize it. The tricky thing about trying to affect a muscle that is entrapping a nerve is to avoid over-stimulating an already sensitized nerve. This is quite difficult, especially because the nerve does not give you immediate feedback the way a muscle does. Tweak the nerve, and you do not know until later. Do exactly the correct approach for the nerve and you won't know until later. Delayed feedback makes working with nerves far more difficult than working with muscles. In addition to treating the scalenes, I also addressed the diaphragm directly. I wasn't sure this would have any real effect, but I wasn't willing to put all my eggs into the scalene basket. This poor guy had suffered enough. We needed the hiccups to stop, and fast, before he and his wife jumped out a window!

I spent about twenty minutes with him the first day, followed by two more daily sessions of about the same duration. Not surprisingly, there was no improvement after the first two sessions. With many conditions, you see a decrease in frequency or intensity, but it is hard to have a less intense hiccup. There aren't really smaller hiccups or bigger ones. While I was hoping that the hiccups would lessen in frequency, this was not a given, either. Since I had no clinical history to go on (I do not specialize in hiccup removal), I was unsure what the time-line and qualities of improvement might be. I could tell that they were a bit discouraged after the third treatment, since no appreciable change had occurred.

When my secretary said that the wife of the guy with hic-cups was on the line, I was sure they were not coming in for the fourth treatment. I was correct, they were not coming in, but not for the reason I feared. After the third session, the hic-cups disappeared, as quickly as they had come. His wife was pretty ecstatic, and I was thrilled. My guess is that they both enjoyed a quiet night's rest for the first time in weeks, a well deserved one at that!

STEP ON IT

L came to see me at the request of one of my students. L is a fit woman whose age I would guess to be around seventy.

"What brings you here?"

"It is my toes; it feels like they are rubbing against each other."

There are times in my practice when I really struggle with the expectations my clients have. I had helped L previously with plantar fascitis and a hip issue, and now she expects help with her toes rubbing against each other. This dilemma was complicated by the fact that she had driven close to two hours to see me. It was too uncomfortable to suggest that she visit her local podiatrist instead since she had driven such a long way for this appointment. What to do?

"Show me what you mean," I said. "Which toes?" (I was stalling for time while trying to come up with a plan.)

She pulled off her socks to reveal very sensitive areas on the little toe and also the great toe, both clearly the result of friction. The greater question was why? Can soft tissue solve this problem? How in the world could I help keep someone's toes from rubbing together?

This is when things started to get a bit (okay, a lot) weird. When I looked at L's toes, it was clear that the fourth toe was pointing towards the little toe, which was the reason for the friction. What a strange sight; the fourth toe was pointing slightly towards the little toe and the second toe was pointing towards the great toe. (Perhaps there was some great family feud brewing here. Maybe an offensive comment made by the third toe, which made both of its neighboring toes point in another direction. It was, perhaps, a scandal of the greatest proportions!)

As I stared at her toes pointing in divergent directions, I asked L to stand up, which loaded the foot. As she went from sitting (nonweight-bearing) to standing (weight-bearing), the slight divergence of her fourth and second toes escalated into a dramatic shift. During weight-bearing, her fourth toe pushed against her little toe and her second toe jammed up to the great toe.

Whenever I have seen such a shift, my first thought was to wonder if I saw that correctly. Was it worse than I thought?

Having L sit again, I watched the toes shift back to their slight misdirection. As she stood, the toes deviated severely, as previously mentioned. I must have had this poor woman go from sitting to standing five times as I observed this distortion intensify with weight-bearing and minimize with sitting. It was fascinating!

The muscles that spread and close the digits of the toes are the lumbricals and the interosseus muscles. Like any other soft-tissue restriction, tightness in a muscle can distort structure. Clearly, her structure (in this case her toes) was distorted. The question is, why did this happen?

The simplest approach to this problem, which she had already tried, was to insert a little spacer to force the toes to be straight. Occasionally this strategy works, but not often. It is similar to a rail next to the gutter in a bowling alley. It will keep the ball from going in the gutter, but you will still get a lousy score if you throw the ball incorrectly.

If the problem is predominately muscular, the tightness in the tissue could pull the toe laterally when the foot is off the ground. In her case, the spread was far worse *in* gravity than *not in* non-gravity. There was a little distortion when she was sitting and I was holding her foot, but the distortion was markedly accentuated during standing.

Distortions in the feet that maximize during weight-bearing point to causes other than soft-tissue tightness. Upon closer examination, I also noticed that L's transverse arch on that foot had fallen significantly relative to the transverse arch on her other foot. Out of gravity, there was no pressure on the arch; in gravity, her arch collapsed. As the transverse arch collapses, the foot widens. Shoes that used to be comfortable now feel a bit too small in the toes, as though a wider shoe is needed. All this fit with L's symptoms and her feeling that her toes were compressed. It did not explain why two toes angled off in divergent directions, but the distortion was clearly worse when she was bearing weight.

Seeing this, I decided to have L wait while I made a quick phone call to a friend named Van who knows exponentially more about foot structure than I do. The running shoe store in which he works has incredibly knowledgeable sales people, and Van is one of their best. Luckily, the store was still open, and L was my last client. I hurried L to my car and we drove over to meet Van before the store closed. As Van fitted and refitted inserts, supports, and shoes, it was fascinating to see L's foot structure change in response to the interventions. After much tweaking and fitting of a metatarsal arch, L's foot finally looked substantially better during weight-bearing. Best of all, she could feel the difference when she walked. Van and I could also see how much more stable her foot was during the gait cycle.

As we drove back to my office, L was thanking me profusely for all my help. I smiled and thought about how little I had actually done. Sometimes, the best way to help unusual cases is to route them to people who know more. The key to serving our clients well is to have clear criteria for knowing when muscular issues are a response to another problem and when soft tissue itself is the cause. In the case of L, I just needed her to step on it to reveal the answer!

The task is . . . not so much to see what no one has yet seen; but to think what nobody has yet thought, about that which everybody sees.

- Ervin Schrödinger

YOU NEVER SEE WHAT YOU DO NOT LOOK FOR

I first saw Mr. W when he popped into my office to see if he could get an appointment. He presented with chronic back pain, most of which was centered at the right low back area. He had had this pain for many years, in fact, as long as he could remember. Mr. W had been to several practitioners in search of relief. The list of people he had seen included numerous MD's, physical therapists, and several local chiropractors. None of these interventions gave him any real relief, so eventually he stopped going. After a while, he would get up the courage to try something else, but that too would fail. He was referred to me by a friend of his who had seen me for back pain.

Upon examination, a possible reason for his back pain became quite clear. When I had Mr. W stand up to look at his structure, his right hip was clearly higher than the left. When measured, the height discrepancy was 11mm superior on the right. This was also evidenced by a discrepancy in his trochanteric heights, PSIS, and ASIS in standing. His right shoulder was 15mm lower than his left, reflecting a compensatory "C" curve in his spine.

"Tell me more about this pain," I asked. "When is it worse?"

"It isn't all that terrible in the morning, just a little fussy when I awaken. It loosens up after about an hour or so. By mid-morning, I feel pretty good. By early afternoon, it begins to intensify. If I sit down for about ten minutes or so, it seems to provide relief. I am good to go for about another hour. Then I need to sit again for another ten minutes. As the afternoon wears on, the sitting doesn't help as much and I have to take more frequent breaks. By the time I go home, I am hurting pretty badly, much more if I have had to be on my feet a lot. I typically have dinner with my wife and relax around the house in the evening, which helps. The next day the cycle starts all over again."

"Come over here and sit on the side of my treatment table."

As Mr. W sat down, I paid particular attention to the reaction of his spine to sitting. When sitting, the "C" curve disappeared. I asked him to stand up again, and the "C" curve reappeared. Sitting a second time, the curve again disappeared.

"What are you looking at?" asked Mr. W.

"I am watching your spine and it is quite fascinating! When you stand, you have one hip that is much higher than the other. Since your spine sits on the pelvis, if the pelvis is unlevel your spine has to compensate. Your spine has a compensatory curve shaped like a "C" when you stand. Here is the cool thing; it disappears when you sit. Your spine goes almost completely straight."

"Oh," he said. "That's great." After hesitating for a bit, he spoke again. "I don't think I understand what that means."

"When you stand, your pelvis is not level so your spine has to compensate. When you sit, you essentially take your lower body out of the picture. The fact that your spine straightens out tells me two things. First, the distortion in your pelvis is likely due to your lower body, such as an anatomically short leg. Second, the fact that your spine straightens up when you sit tells me that your spine is quite resilient. That is great news! Often, even if the lower body is the cause, the spine stays distorted simply because it is so used to being so. Your spine goes back to normal when the forces distorting it are removed. That will likely mean that if we correct the lower body distortion, your spine is going to like this a lot."

"Does that explain why I get relief from sitting? Maybe that is why the back pain is worse when I have to be on my feet for long periods of time."

"You are exactly right," I replied. "Who am I to say, but it sure looks like you could have an anatomically short left leg. It is not my place to say so, but I know what I would do if I were you. You might want to consider going to Walgreens and getting an insert for your left shoe. Just get an inexpensive flat full insert and see how you respond. I don't want you to notice much of anything except maybe a bit less back pain. After a bit, we will add another insert and then when it is about the right height, we can have a podiatrist make an orthotic for you."

"I am OK with just getting the orthotic right away if you want", replied Mr. W.

"I'd rather you not do that," I replied. (Mr. W and I have a mutual friend who is a podiatrist.) If you go to see Dr. M, he will likely make you an orthotic that corrects for the full discrepancy all at once. There is a risk in doing so for two reasons. One is that it is a heck of a change for your body. It may be uncomfortable and I'd rather take the long route. The second reason is that I may be wrong about how connected your back pain is to your leg length discrepancy." I'd rather you spend $12 to find out whether I am correct that have you spend $400 only to find out I am wrong."

"Do you mean that you are not sure I have a leg length discrepancy? You seemed pretty sure."

"I am reasonably sure you do. The bigger question is whether or not that is really connected to your back pain. Think about it. The MD's you saw found something on an image and treated you for that condition. The physical therapists probably found you have weak muscles and gave you specific exercises. The chiropractors you saw probably found misalignment issues in your back and treated such. Each practitioner found something they deemed wrong and treated it. Each diagnosis was probably correct; it just didn't have anything to do with your pain. You can't really even call the treatment a failure, since they may have corrected the issue they found. The bigger problem is relevance. These people all fixed existing problems; it's just that these problems didn't have a lot to do with your back pain. I don't want to make the same mistake as they did. Even though this unlevel pelvis seems like a really good bet, there is no guarantee. Let's try the least invasive and least expensive route first."

In less than a month, Mr. W had undergone quite a change. His back pain was substantially improved for the first time in memory. To say he was pleased is an understatement. I did treat him a couple times, but really the inserts were probably the biggest reason for his improvement. His custom orthotic from our podiatrist friend was comfortable and a good investment.

"I just have one question," Mr. W asked at the end of his last session. "If the hip height thing was so obvious, why the heck didn't anyone else see this?"

"Well, the real answer is that you never see what you do not look for. Most disciplines do not acknowledge that leg length discrepancies are important or related to back pain. Some think that even a half inch difference in length is purely cosmetic. Walk around for a day with one shoe on and one shoe off and see how cosmetic it feels! If you don't think it important, there is no reason to look for it. Obviously for you, the discrepancy was at the heart of your pain."

I still see Mr. W in social settings and his back has continued to be substantially better. I always savor his warm smile and firm handshake that conveys his gratitude.

IT HURTS WHEN YOU WHAT?

She was just about to get on my treatment able when I stopped her.

"It hurts when you what?" I asked.

"If I bend sideways to the right," she replied. "It is much worse if I raise my arms up in the air, but it hurts even if my arms are by my side."

I stood there with my mouth open, trying to process what I was seeing. Miss N was referred to me because of a rectus femoris / hip capsule issue. In fact, she had just had a steroid shot a few days earlier into her left hip joint because the doctor was concerned about a possible teres ligament tear. Miss M is a dancer, and a very good one, who has not been able to dance for the last couple months. Nothing is worse than watching your peers do what you really want to be doing; she had been away from the stage for far too long.

I had met Miss M for a few minutes one week ago. She had approached me after a lecture I gave and asked if I might take a look at her left hip. I did so and found her psoas attachment and rectus femoris to be quite sensitive. She had explained the litany of health care providers that she had seen and every one of them had a slightly different version of what was wrong with her hip. I found sensitivity in the periarticular tissue and thought it was reasonable to explore that. Now, she was describing a movement that has nothing to do with her hip.

I asked her to bend sideways repeatedly as I watched, looking for some kind of clue. I needed a way to confirm and disconfirm the rectus femoris as the culprit. Sliding a chair under her bent knee seemed to answer the call. Standing with the left knee bent at 90 degrees puts the rectus femoris on a prestretch. The psoas is unaffected by the position of the knee, only the position of the hip. If it was the rectus femoris, the pain should be worse, and we would have found our culprit.

"How is that?" I asked as she bent to the right with her left knee flexed.

"Maybe a little better. I can't really tell, but I think it is easier."

"What? You have got to be kidding?" I was incredulous. I just stared at her blankly.

"Wrong answer, huh?" she said wryly. I just stared.

Why in the world would it be slightly better? Clearly, the rectus femoris was not the source of the problem. I positioned her hip carefully into hip extension as we did the same movement to implicate the psoas. I was propping her hip up on my treatment stool, which was just a little too high, elevating the pelvis on the left side. Hip extension, not spinal extension, seemed to have no appreciable effect on her pain. If I took away the stool, which lowered her pelvis on that side, the pain was much worse. The path forward suddenly became clearer.

I asked Miss M to lie on the table face up and I slowly began to examine her oblique muscles and the rectus abdominus for trigger point activity. I found several taut bands, each of which was remarkably tender. Just as I was about to explain how important it is to replicate symptoms, her face lit up. She excitedly told me that she could feel the referral from the spot in her abdomen that I was treating right to the front of her hip, which replicated her pain. Importantly, I also felt the classic taut band and nodule, the tissue texture that is the hallmark of trigger point activity.

After a few minutes of Precision Neuromuscular Therapy treatment, I asked Miss M to stand up and repeat the side-bending movement. She did so, her face was beaming. She explained that there was no pain in right lateral flexion and it did not matter if her arms were up or down. We were making progress!

Finding trigger points in the oblique also explained why the pain was worse when she bent to the right side with her arms up in the air. Having the arms in the air stretches the oblique muscle, whereas putting her arms down relaxed the oblique.

This was all wonderful, but it did not explain one little detail. Miss M also happened to mention that her left hip felt restricted in external rotation. I had measured her hip external rotation and indeed, it was restricted relative to the right hip. What could be the source of this? External restrictions of the hip are very uncommon for a dancer. Was there a connection to the oblique? Why hadn't this shown up with the earlier hip extension testing?

I again had Miss M stand with her bent left knee resting on my treatment stool. When I asked her to do hip extension, I noticed something I probably missed earlier; she pivoted her femur into internal rotation as she did hip extension. Clever! To take stretch off the tensor fascia lata (TFL), which is stretched in hip extension, she unknowingly created an internal rotation of the femur to reduce the stretch. Having her sustain hip extension, I pivoted the stool slightly to create external rotation and the stretch was too much for her.

"Wow! I can't believe that little pivot makes such a difference!" Miss M exclaimed.

Having her lie on the table again, I carefully treated the TFL, which resolved quite nicely. This absolutely astounded Miss M because friends of hers had aggressively treated this area, and it never had become less tender. Why did the sensitivity on the TFL lessen so quickly now?

The answer is in the relationship of the TFL to the referral area from the oblique muscles. Trigger points in an area of referral from another source are likely to reform again, unless the primary source is neutralized. Instead of treating these stubborn areas aggressively, look for a distant referral source. In the case of Miss M, it worked perfectly. I went to a dance performance that Ms M was in about seven weeks later. She was superb!

☙❧

WAIT, DON'T HANG UP!

"Wait, don't hang up. What did you say?" I couldn't quite believe my ears.

"I said that I understand if you don't think you can help me. Every doctor I have seen thinks I'm nuts. I guess this thing just can't be helped. I can at least stop the ringing in my ear for awhile by pushing up on my jaw. Thanks for listening anyway."

"Whoa! That's what I thought you said, the part about pushing on your jaw to make the ringing stop. You can do that?" I asked.

"Yes," she replied. "Isn't that weird?"

"I want to see you Monday!" I exclaimed. "I think there is a chance we can solve this! Forget what I said earlier."

Let me back up just a bit. Mrs. B had been a client of one of my students who was seeing him for relief of neck pain. During the session, she mentioned to him that she experienced ringing in her ears, which had lasted for over a year, and it was highly annoying. She thought it may have begun after a car accident but wasn't exactly sure the two were related.

As the ringing got worse, she sought help from physicians, but the pursuit of an answer had been frustrating. After many hearing tests, otoscope examinations, and neural exams, she was no farther along than before. She had even been referred to a TMJ specialist who was unfamiliar with any connection between temporomandibular issues and ringing in the ear. (Has this person been reading the literature? It was hard to suppress my surprise and dismay.)

While I appreciated the referral, often students refer cases to me that cannot be helped by soft-tissue therapy. The client may have a combination of post-polio, fibromyalgia, and focal dystonia, and the student wants to know what muscle to treat to solve it. It isn't that easy.

Every symptom may have multiple causes. Ringing in the ears is extremely complex. There are many possible reasons, many which are not in the realm of soft-tissue treatment. For instance, kidney dysfunction will cause ringing in the ear. So will prolonged exposure to loud noises and a host of other conditions. Since Mrs. B was going to have to drive two hours for appointments with me, I didn't want to start working with her unless I had a reasonable chance of helping her problem.

In that light, I explained the multiple possible causes of tinnitus and how I was hesitant to have her commit to such an effort to see me without assurance that the work had a reasonable chance of success. Discouraging her from coming was probably the right choice, until she ended the conversation with the comment about stopping the ear ringing by pushing up on the jaw.

Of all the possible causes that I mentioned to her, none of them would be influenced by pushing superiorly on the mandible. Your kidneys do not care if you push on the mandible or not and tinnitus from loud noises doesn't care.

Mrs. B's ability to stop the ringing by pressing on the jaw revealed that the source of the ringing was mechanical in nature since a mechanical act affected it. This was huge!!! This meant the likelihood of me helping her was now exceedingly good, rather than a long shot.

Encouraged by this, I saw Mrs. B for three treatments. Through careful work to her mandibular and aural area, she has noticed a significant reduction in the ringing for the first time. I was encouraged by my own clinical experience in treating tinnitus as well as relying on the literature. In a study by Carina A.C. Rocha and Tanit Ganz Sanchez from the University of São Paulo School of Medicine, the researchers looked at 94 patients with tinnitus and examined trigger points in the masseter, splenius capitis, sternocleidomastoid, and temporalis muscles and found that 72 percent of the 94 patients with tinnitus had relevant trigger points. Mrs. B also had relevant trigger points, mostly in the masseter and temporalis muscles. The researchers also found that 60 percent of the group experienced a lessening of their tinnitus after treatment of the trigger points.

The researchers also looked at another aspect: correlating pain on one side of the upper body with the tinnitus. A strong correlation existed between the side of the worst tinnitus and the side of the upper body in the most pain. This was also true for Mrs. B. It is extremely important to know the research and be able to convey it to our clients.

Mrs. B is not unusual in one respect: because the people treating her could not connect all her symptoms, they did not believe her. When looking at an array of symptoms, any clinician must decide what is relevant and what is not. The deciding factor is the knowledge base of the healthcare provider. Three skills are crucial: listen carefully to all details, hear what the client describes as connected, and know the literature.

I have often thought that the greatest service I have provided to clients is connecting their symptoms—moving from chaos to a place where people understand the context of their experience. I often hear a sigh of relief as I show the client the literature that connects presenting but confusing symptoms. Mrs. B was no exception. She was relieved to know she wasn't really nuts after all, there was an answer, and I put my finger on it. Mrs. B continued to improve very nicely over three sessions. I'm just glad she didn't hang up. So is she!

MOBILITY AND STABILITY

"That is very strange. I don't understand why I can't do that."

From across the room, I could hear the concern in her voice as all of the participants in the class were working away. As I worked through the room toward the two therapists, I could see the confusion in her face.

The instructions I had given to the class were very simple. I asked them to measure the capability for each to perform humeral abduction, which should be about 165°. What these two therapists who were partnered had noticed was striking. If the young lady who was the "client" (call her "M") lifted one arm in abduction, her maximum ability was 90°. This was also true on the other arm, which was also capable of only 90°. While limited, this may not be that unusual. What was remarkable was that for some reason, this young woman experimented with raising both arms at once, which resulted in flawless motion on both sides to about 165°. What she could not understand was why she could not rise beyond 90° on either side individually, but if she lifted both sides simultaneously; her arms went to full abduction.

124

I must admit that I hoped my face did not show that I was just as confused as she. This made no sense whatever. Her arms clearly were capable of full abduction, so no joint issues could be present. How could it be a muscular issue if the muscles were capable of creating and allowing the motion, albeit only when both sides contracted at once? What was it about bilateral contraction that enabled her to raise her arms to full range?

It is at these moments when all the time spent studying anatomy pays off. Watching her abduct her arms, the explanation finally hit me. I tried a little experiment to confirm my hypothesis.

"Before you abduct your left arm, I want you to push your right arm against me as though you were trying to abduct it," I said.

As I held her right arm tightly to her body while she pushed against me, she easily lifted her left arm up to 165°. She looked at me in confusion as she lifted her left arm again and again into full abduction. To make a point, I did the same thing to her other side. If I resisted her abduction on the left, she could easily raise her right arm into full abduction. She was about to explode with curiosity.

"Let me show you something that explains your situation, but will also teach you a very important lesson about functional anatomy," I said.

I took her partner therapist and asked that person to hold her right arm at 90° of abduction. Firmly, I pressed into her arm, resisting her abductors. I then placed M's hand on the mid-scapular area and asked her to palpate where she felt contraction. M responded that she felt very strong contraction on the left side of her friend's back along the spinal erectors and scapular stabilizers. This made perfect sense; when you place weight out on the lever arm, something must contract to stabilize that weight. In M, this was not happening as the stabilizers, for whatever reason, were not firing. Raising both arms together created its own stabilization, i.e. it activated both sides at once, fixing the stabilization problem.

To demonstrate a correction, I treated M's left scapular and spinal stabilizers with a rather vigorous up-regulation technique. Immediately following, she was able to raise her right arm into full abduction. Doing the same treatment on the right side allowed her to raise her left arm into full abduction. She smiled and slowly shook her head in disbelief.

The lesson here is that any muscle contraction can do its job _only_ if there is a stable base from which to operate. If that base is not stable, the brain will shut down the muscle contraction to prevent injury. Muscle shortness/tightness is not the only reason for lack of range of motion. Mobility and stability are forever linked.

QUESTION EVERYTHING

Mrs. H, a spritely woman in her mid-sixties, presented herself to my office on a cool March morning. Looking a little frustrated, yet hopeful, she relayed her story.

"I have been struggling with my right shoulder for almost two years now. I am an artist, painting with watercolors, and my shoulder really affects my painting. It has progressively gotten worse over time. At this point, I cannot lift it higher than this (She lifted her arm to about 70 degrees of forward flexion and about the same in abduction).

I did go see my doctor about two months ago, and she took an x-ray of my shoulder. She said that the likely cause of my pain is a bone spur and that surgery is needed to remove the spur. My friend, Ron, has seen you and suggested I consult you first, as you have helped him and many others avoid surgery or a life on medication. I'd like to do anything I can to avoid surgery."

At this point, I had a sinking feeling that this may not go well. If any therapeutic approach garners success, it always seems that the second step is overestimation of what is possible.

"Let me explain something. If the X-ray shows a bone spur under the acromial shelf, the spur acts like a thorn sticking downwards. Every time you raise your arm, that thorn is shredding the tendon of a muscle underneath it. Usually, by the time they try the repair, the tendon is shredded into pieces. The more you lift your arm, the more you shred the tendon."

"But I want to do everything possible to avoid surgery; I just don't believe in it," she stated.

"The bone spur doesn't really care if you believe in it or not. It just is. Each time you raise your arm above 90 degrees, the spur comes in contact with the tendon. Soft tissue work is unlikely to change that."

Mrs. H looked pretty disappointed, and I felt bad for not having the answer that she wanted to hear. I suggested that as long as she was here, we should take a look at the soft-tissue anyway. I did this mostly to help her feel attended to since I did not feel I could solve her problem.

As expected, I found sensitivity in numerous muscles of the shoulder girdle, concentrating on none of them in particular, at this point. As she was talking about her artwork, I happened to lift her arm into full flexion and abduction. I think I did this absolutely reflexively, more by default than by design. She kept speaking passionately about her artwork, not responding at all to the movements I was doing. It took a moment for me to register the full significance of what just transpired. Stopping the treatment, I asked her to sit.

As she sat up, I passively moved her arm into abduction and moved it in multiple positions. No negative response from her at all.

"Do you remember what I said earlier about the bone spur? Everything I said about the spur and the tendon was correct, but I am not sure that applies to your shoulder. Think about it. If the bone spur is the source of your pain, why isn't it painful when I lift your arm? The spur should still be coming in contact with the tendon. It should hurt you now, but it doesn't. (I was holding her arm at more than 90 degrees of abduction) The pain exists only when you actively lift the arm, which means it is a contractile problem; one due to muscles complaining about either length or strength. Lift your arm again, slowly if possible, and tell me where you feel restriction."

She did this and pointed to the underside of her arm, in the area of the latissimus and teres muscles. Horrified, I wondered why in the world I didn't do this simple test first. It would have clarified the problem right away, pointing me away from the bone spur as the source of pain. I do this with everyone else; how could I overlook something so simple?

The answer to this question is that I, like the physician, got sucked down the path provided by the diagnostic image. Just because there is a problem or pathology on the screen does not mean that this pathology is the source of pain. In the case of Mrs. H, this was indeed true. In just three careful thirty minute treatments she was able to lift her arm without pain. The impediment to great problem solving is often the assumptions we accept as true, whether or not they are confirmed by what the client presents to us. The table lesson from Mrs. H is: assume nothing, question everything, and the final answer should address *every* facet of their symptom presentation and history.

Our doubts are our traitors and make us lose the good we oft might win, by fearing the attempt.

Shakespeare

I HATE GOING TO BED

"You what?" I asked.

"I hate going to bed at night. I just dread it. All day long I feel essentially fine, but oh, when night falls and I try to get some rest, the suffering begins. It doesn't matter if I lie on my right side or my let side, both produce the same pain."

Mrs. S had that look of dread on her face when someone knows that discomfort is looming. Clearly, she had been at her wits end about this pain, certainly understandable when sleep is something to be feared. To her, night was a curse. As long as she moved around, all was well. When she tried to get some sleep, the pain was unleashed in full force!

The particulars of her case were quite interesting. The pain she described was a pain going down the leg all the way to the lateral side of the ankle. Like many people, due to the nature of the pain, she had a hard time localizing the discomfort. When I pressed her, she clarified that the pain was in the front of the thigh, going down to the knee and then diverting a bit laterally and streaming down the side of the anterior tibialis. This pain was more of a deep ache, something that was very uncomfortable but not location specific.

Mrs. S had an activity level that few people could match. A woman in her sixties, she had completed many marathons and half marathons. Instead of running fifteen to eighteen miles at a time, she has cut back to running no more than five miles at a time.

"Did you cut back your mileage because of pain?" I inquired.

"That's the thing, running has never bothered me. I cut back only because I think that I should and that people tell me that running is probably the reason for the pain. People have told me to stop running, but it never bothers me when I run or even anytime after a run. A couple of friends tried to get me to stretch a lot more, but it actually hurt worse when I started stretching my thigh more intensely. Other than that, the only time the pain bothers me is at night. Except for when I walk up stairs, I never feel the pain during the day.

"Stairs?" I asked.

"Yes, I do feel discomfort when I have to walk up stairs. We have just a few in our house, so I don't really notice it much. I did notice that during a visit to Chicago, we went to some buildings that had a lot of stairs and the pain was a bit like what I feel at night."

"Did you feel the pain going up or coming down? This is very important."

"Only going up, never going down stairs."

At this point, the options for Mrs. S seemed to be pretty clear. I ran through a checklist of what might be the source of her problem. I took her hip and ran it through a complete range of motion assessment. Her range seemed excellent in all planes, making it extremely unlikely that there were low level arthritic changes in the joint. (Low level arthritic issues are worse at night, better with use.)

The only plausible solution was a trigger point in her gluteus minimus muscle. The referral pattern is almost exactly as she described, and it seemed like a perfect match- Except for one little detail, the nocturnal only pain. Why wouldn't the pain be aggravated by an activity that stresses the muscle, such as single leg standing? Single leg standing would be involved in going up stairs, and it would also be implicated in running even more. (Do they make nocturnal trigger points?) Hoping for the easy answer, I thoroughly checked every millimeter of her gluteus minimus. While I found tenderness, (as I would on everyone) not one spot replicated her symptoms. Great idea, albeit clearly off the mark.

"Let's try something. I am going to put your thigh on a stretch. Tell me when you feel a slight pull in the front of your thigh." I had her in a lateral recumbent position, stretching the rectus femoris muscle. Once she felt the stretch, I asked her to move her head into extension while I was very careful not to allow any change in the position of her hip or knee. Moving her head into extension, she remarked that the stretch she had previously felt in her thigh immediately disappeared. Moving her head into flexion made the stretch in her anterior thigh much worse.

"That's weird," she said with a curious voice.

"More than weird, it is the answer to the whole problem. I am pretty sure I know the source of your pain and where to go from here. I also know why stretching made it worse and why the problem only happens at night. It is very likely that you have a problem with one of the nerves that runs in the front of your thigh. Nerve pain is worse at night, due to lack of movement, as (axoplasmic) fluid inside the nerve slows down. Movement reestablishes that flow, which is why if you awaken and walk for awhile, symptoms disappear. (She was nodding in approval at this point). The reason your head movement makes the stretch worse is that when you move your head into extension, you slacken the nerve, while the muscle length never changes. Essentially, what you feel as a pull in the thigh is a neural sensation, not muscular tightness.

The other issue is that the strategy for addressing the muscle (rectus femoris) through stretching is the wrong thing to do for the nerve. What helps one is exactly what will irritate the other. Show me how you were stretching the muscle."

At this point, Mrs. S got up and did the typical standing stretch for the rectus femoris, but as she reached back to pull her heel to her chest, I noticed that she had her head in full cervical flexion. Cervical flexion puts maximum stretch on the nerve, a great way to further irritate it. This is why the increased stretching made her problem worse. A rectus femoris issue and a femoral nerve issue *feel* exactly the same. One symptom with two very different causes and two very different, almost opposite, solutions.

What followed my explanation has happened so often in my career, yet it always amazes me. Mrs. S revealed that this problem had indeed happened once before, about three years ago. During that episode, she was desperate for a solution, just as she had been with this bout of pain. The first few doctors asked her to discontinue running for six weeks, which she did. After weeks of giving up what she loved, the pain was unchanged. What followed were numerous MRI's and other imaging studies and then finally a nerve conduction test, which implicated the femoral nerve (Who knew?). Once having a diagnosis, no one seemed to know what to do about it. She finally gave up on the medical pursuit and started easy running again. The pain disappeared on its own until now. (I find it amazing that she could forget to tell me this previous history, but in her mind it was inconsequential as the pain went away in spite of the care, not because of anything medically that was done. Besides, she was in no hurry to repeat the nerve conduction test anytime soon. (Who can blame her?)

During the session, I released the entire path of the femoral nerve with careful fascial work. The point of the fascial work is to release any possible adhesion that could be tethering the nerve, restricting it from achieving full movement capability. We don't normally think about the effect of movement on nerves, but any movement that requires lengthening of a muscle also affects a nerve. For example, when you bend forward at the waist, the nerves in your back and legs must have enough slack in them to allow the movement to happen. The muscles must lengthen, but the nerves must also allow the motion to occur. If the nerves don't have enough slack, the resultant feeling from neural restriction is indistinguishable from muscular tightness. Again, this is problematic because the solution for muscular tightness (direct stretching) irritates the nerve. The original test I did for Mrs. S (moving her neck to affect the stretch she felt in her thigh), was a way to test the nerve by stretching it. At the end of the session, this original test was no longer positive, meaning that moving her head had no effect on the stretch she felt in her thigh.

At that point, I could see that Mrs. S was quite intrigued by the whole endeavor. As someone who had multiple massages before, she was used to massage therapists digging in her tissue to, well, to do what was never exactly clear. The idea was to get in there and get "it". The nature of the "it" the therapists were after was never really clear. In this case, clear results were made without pain and without struggle. I could see the look of perplexity on her face; she was still expecting a battle between her leg and my thumb at some point, something at least a little more dramatic than what we had done.

"OK, I see that the movement no longer bothers me. I can't say I absolutely understand this as to how it happened, but the results are clear. What do I need to do from here?"

"First, don't do any more of the stretching you were doing. Second, let me show you a simple movement for encouraging the nerve to glide freely."

"Can I run?" she asked pleadingly.

"Has running ever made this worse?" I asked.

"No."

"Then there is no reason to stop, but I want to you to continue to limit runs to less than seven miles. What I am really looking for is the cessation of pain at night. When the nocturnal pain stops, we have accomplished stage one. A victory on stage two will be when you do not notice any pain when going up stairs. Stage three, the final stage, will be complete when you don't notice pain ever."

I sent Mrs. S off, hoping that I was on the right course. I did get an email from her about three weeks later. At first, she had a hard time doing the neural movements I gave her because they did not enlist symptoms, but she did them anyway. After two weeks, she began sleeping through the night. This was a big breakthrough for her, since nocturnal pain was her main complaint. Her running continued to be fine and she was slowly increasing her mileage, with no effect on her pain. Going up stairs was only occasionally painful, and, that too faded after seven weeks. Best of all, she no longer fears going to bed!

SECTION FOUR: COMMUNICATION

In any relationship, the ability to communicate effectively is the key to success. The relationship between client and massage therapist is one in which effective communication is essential and also fraught with peril. The ability of the therapist to communicate what is going to happen and why will put the client at ease. Clients often do not realize how essential their experience of the treatment is to the therapist. Clients often feel as though the therapist can ascertain everything they need to know by palpating the tissue.

Effective communication is essential to success in the treatment room.

The beginning of knowledge is the discovery of something we do not understand.

Frank Herbert

LOST

Mrs. G entered my treatment room, having seen me several times previously for a shoulder issue. She is an artist and while it is questionable that her work caused the shoulder pain, it clearly affects it. For the record, her pain has improved tremendously since she first visited the office. It went from something that she thought she had to endure to a minor annoyance. That is a substantial change, one that I sometimes have to remind a frustrated client about when the last 10-15% of pain is slow to disappear.

As I do with every client, I wanted an update before we started to work.

"Well, it is still there. I mean not like it was though. But I don't mean to sound like it is almost gone; I am aware of it often. It can happen when I am in my studio, although it doesn't always do that. Actually, it can happen at any time. Wait, I know you are going to ask me with what motion it hurts worst. (At this point, she went though several shoulder motions, none of which produced the symptoms). Well, even though it is not doing it now, it usually hurts if I reach forward like this, but sometimes if I reach backward. It really does come and go."

There was kind of an awkward silence as I did not respond to any of this; I couldn't think of how to respond.

"That didn't make a lot of sense did it?" Mrs. G said sheepishly.

"Actually, it didn't," I heard myself reply.

At that moment, I was transported to another time, about several years earlier.

Once when I was teaching a seminar, I agreed to see someone who was in pain for demonstration purposes. (This is not something I often do, for a number of reasons.) The main reason I agreed to see the person was that the therapist, who was one of my students, was bringing this client. The therapist was not taking the seminar but was willing to drive the client to the seminar site for an evaluation. With insights gleaned from my assessment, the client would have follow-up care from her therapist. This seemed ideal for everyone.

I saw this client at the end of class and invited the students who wanted to stay and watch to do so. I recall that all thirty of them stayed and sat around the periphery of the room. The therapist decided to let the client relay her story to me; any input from the therapist could be given later.

The client, a woman in her mid-thirties, was clearly suffering and was anxious to relay her story to the class. She was remarkably forthright in speaking to everyone, not shy with such a large audience. She spoke about the pain, how pervasive it was and the impact it had had on her life. She spoke about her experiences with health-care, not much of which was good. Her account of how the pain had affected her family was gut-wrenching. She described attributes of the pain, describing in detail the nuances of its qualities.

At this point, I got a bit distracted. Out of the corner of my eye, I could see my class shifting in their chairs, exchanging glances, and looking pretty uncomfortable. Was it just the length of time that was affecting them? The explanation from the client had gone on for perhaps fifteen to eighteen minutes.

Come to think of it, I was feeling uncomfortable too. Looking for a space to interrupt her, I signaled to the client that I had a question. She hesitated long enough to let me speak; allowing me to share what had been bugging me for the last ten minutes or so.

"I'm lost." There, I said it. The client looked horrified.

"I hate to say this, but I am truly lost about something. The account of the pain and how it has affected your life is remarkable. However, you keep referring to the pain as 'it'. I have no idea if the 'it' you are referring to is a pain in your little toe, your back, or your finger."

Out of the corner of my eye, I could see students almost falling off the chairs that held them. Everyone was glancing at each other, and I knew I had struck a nerve. What was bothering them, and bothering me, was that everyone felt like they were the only one in the room who had missed something obvious. Each of us felt like we missed the most crucial, yet simple detail: what hurts? The student's previous glances and shuffling were an effort to see if anyone else looked lost. We were all lost, but none of us had missed anything.

The client was absolutely stunned for ten to fifteen seconds. I could see her mind processing, thinking either this guy is a real dunce, or he has a serious hearing problem. After a bit of silence, a very sad look emerged on her face.

"Oh my gosh, I can't believe that I never told you where I hurt. I never realized this until just now, but I guess I do refer to the pain as though it is right here next to me and visible to all. This pain has been so much a part of my life that I do not see it as separate. How sad is that?"

This session sparked a wonderful class discussion the next morning on the pervasiveness of pain and also on communicating well with a client. People in pain, such as this client, live with the pain every moment. When something is that much a part of your life, it is difficult to articulate the qualities and nuances of something so close. Our job as therapists, like a good detective, is to help the client find words to describe the experience. Adding to the problem is fact that the English language lacks an appropriate vocabulary of words to describe pain, and our job is even tougher.

All this flashed through my mind as my client sheepishly stood there after admitting that everything she told me was conflicting and not helpful.

"You're right, I said. "I'm lost. Let's start over and see if we can ferret out more details."

Lost. Even though the word and the situation it represents sound quite negative, I would postulate that there are two kinds of lost. One is to be so hopelessly adrift that recovery does not seem possible. The other is that moment when you first realize you are off-course. The quicker you realize that moment, the better. Becoming hopelessly wayward is usually a product of assuming that you are on course, even when the data around you conflicts with that idea. Like a GPS system, we have to uplink as often as possible to see if *where we are and where we think we are* happen to be the same. In the therapy room, the uplink means checking in with the client as often and as clearly as possible.

We read the world wrong and say that it deceives us.

- Rabindranath Tagore

RUNAWAY MIND SYNDROME

To further illustrate the value of communication, I'd like to share with you the following story that happened several years ago.

I was scheduled to teach a seminar at a particular school that was mostly for their alumni and a few current students. The flyer the school had distributed listed the class as starting at the time I usually do registration, which meant everyone showed up more than a half hour early. My flight was delayed and by the time I walked in the door, the room was already filled with people in their seats. Nothing is quite as uncomfortable as having people watch your every move while setting up equipment. Although somewhat awkwardly, I set everything up and was ready to go in a few minutes.

As I began (with my credibility a bit diminished for being tardy and my adrenaline ramped up from the travel), I sought to establish rapport with my audience. Since I was teaching some pretty cerebral information, I tried to intersperse humor through the process.

I felt this group and I were connecting very well, except for one person way in the back. This person wasn't just in the back; she was in a separate small room at the very end of this seminar room. Sitting at a desk, she was not exactly facing me, but facing forward at the desk. If she was an administrator in the school, perhaps she was getting some work done while I was lecturing. Taking attendance? Taking notes on my lecture? Why wouldn't she join us?

The room was packed with people; each time I tried to get a clear view of the lone person in the adjacent room, my view was blocked by a student. If I shifted left, a student would also shift to block my view. In the goofiest of circumstances, I could never work myself to a position with a clear view of this mystery person in the back. What limited view I did have made clear this person did not respond in the least to any of my humor nor to anything I said. As a speaker, this began to wear on me. Had I said something offensive? Perhaps that line I thought was funny was taken as an offense. I knew I shouldn't have said that, but everyone else thought it was humorous. What if she was from one of the governing bodies that issue approval for continuing education credits? Wow, if they pull my certification because of one comment, I am dead in the water.

Finally, during a break, I decided that direct engagement was the only reasonable strategy. I worked my way through the crowd of people, heading towards the little room in the back, trying to say something to everyone who stopped me with questions. I was determined to engage this menacing person before the break was over. Finally, when I moved closer to the back of the room, my eyes fell upon the figure that had so troubled me for the last hour. Strangely, however, her gaze refused to meet mine. Even with me approaching her, the snub continued.

Then, the reality of the situation hit me like a brick falling from a roof. The woman, the one I had pegged for an IRS auditor, Homeland Security agent, or who-knows-what, was an anatomical mannequin! Are you kidding me? In my defense (I am reaching a bit here, but work with me on this), the school had her dressed up in a normal outfit, posed at the desk in a quite natural position. Skin color, clothes, position, everything was pretty darn natural (unless you actually looked closely).

One evening, the following week, I complimented my wife on how lovely she looked. Her reply was,

"This from a guy who can't tell a mannequin from a real person?"

The outrageous stories concocted by the mind are amazing. We can run screaming down the path of our imagination, only to forget to check in with what is actually real. Clients can exhibit runaway mind syndrome when they assign faulty meaning to pain. Therapists can exhibit runaway mind syndrome when they latch on to a particular belief system as the unified source of every client's pain. Once we make up our mind, we notice little that contradicts our belief or story. We see only that which confirms our ideas and ignore that which negates them. (This is an error in logic called confirmation bias.) We have to be extremely careful to take in every detail possible and keep an open mind as to the meaning of what we observe.

Addendum: I shared this story with one of my friends, who could not resist sharing his runaway mind story with me. I found the story a perfect representation of the runaway mind and hilarious to boot!

A few years ago this man and his wife were travelling in a southern state and stopped for lunch at a casual restaurant and bar. While sitting at the booth with his wife, he could not help but notice that every time he looked up, several people were staring at him. He continued eating his lunch, but couldn't resist looking up more often. Each time he did, he saw people staring at him. Growing more and more agitated, he mentioned to his wife how uncomfortable he was.

"Haven't these people ever seen a Jewish couple before? What is their deal?" he implored.

His wife encouraged him to relax and finish lunch, but the tension became too much. Throwing cash on the table, he stood up from the booth and announced he could not take this anymore; it was time to leave. As he turned to face the booth where he and his wife were sitting, he happened to notice, perched on a shelf directly above their booth, a large television silently broadcasting a sporting event.

"Oh," he said with embarrassment as he slid back in the booth to finish his lunch.

I SHOULD HAVE COME HERE FIRST

"You have had daily headaches for months? Wow. That has to make life very difficult," I stated.

"You have no idea. I have a very busy and demanding job, which I also happen to enjoy very much. Between that and the demands of taking care of my child and trying to spend some time with my husband, these headaches really get in the way of enjoying life. My life is busy, but really good except for these damn headaches."

Mrs. R had been referred to me from a physical therapist. This PT is very skilled, and I wanted to know what they had been doing.

"Well, she has really helped me think about my posture and functionality at work," said R. "I have found that to be really helpful. I have really improved my posture since we first started working. She and I have worked really hard at improving my daily routine; I am using my body better, but it really has not improved the headache situation. That is pretty crappy because the headaches are the reason I went to her in the first place and I didn't expect to improve my comfort at work. I have benefited in ways I did not expect, but the original problem remains the same."

"Why did you see her in the first place? Who referred you?"

"My primary care physician referred me to physical therapy. I told the doctor about my headaches and she suggested physical therapy. I told her about my headaches and that nothing had helped so far."

"So far? You had done something else, then?"

"Yes, I had gone to a chiropractor. He saw some stuff on the x-ray that he didn't like, and I had multiple treatments to correct it. Like the physical therapy, I noticed improvement in ways I did not expect. My neck was more mobile, but it did not have any effect on the headaches. That is when I went to my doctor and got the physical therapy referral."

"Show me exactly where you feel the headaches. Better yet, do you have a headache now?"

"Sure do, as always. I feel it here (She pressed on the back of her neck at about C3/4), and then it radiates up my head and to my temple. The headache is almost always on the same side."

At that point, I had Mrs. R lie on her side on my treatment table. I slowly and carefully began to examine the semispinalis capitis with a pincer palpation, looking for trigger points that might replicate her symptoms.

"There, right there! That's my headache!"

This is exactly what I was hoping to hear. At this point, I explained to Mrs. R about trigger points and how they refer sensation to distal areas, essentially "call-forwarding" for pain. Since she already had the referred pain experience, all I had to do was validate for her what she already felt. I retrieved the Travel and Simons book <u>Myofascial Pain and Dysfunction</u> from my library and showed her the referral pattern illustrated in the book.

"What you feel when I press on one of these trigger points is what thousands of other people have felt. In fact, this process is based on the work of a doctor named Kellgren, who published his ideas in the 1930s. Kellgren injected a tissue irritant into specific points of the body and created reproducible symptoms in people who had no symptoms previously. He could create a referred sensation via injection and most people would get the same pattern of referral. His ideas originated from a doctor in France in the mid 1800s. Kellgren's work got absolutely no notice until about 1950 when the person who wrote <u>Myofascial Pain and Dysfunction</u> stumbled onto Kellgren's writings and developed them further. Remember, the "x" spot and the referral pattern doesn't just mean that some people have experienced this before. The original methodology was that these symptoms could be replicated and created in people who had no pain to begin with. These referral patterns are not the only ones possible. It simply means that if you inject 100 people in the same place, most of them are going to feel the same thing. Scientifically, that is a very strong argument."

Mrs. R was clearly both amazed and also had that look of validation one gets when you realize you are not the only person in the world to experience something.

"Wow, I'm not nuts! It just amazes me that you can press a spot in my neck and perfectly recreate my headache. Even more so, knowing that this is known and others have had the same experience is kind of comforting. When you have sought treatment with several people and it doesn't work, it makes you wonder if the pain is all in your head. That you can intensify the pain with by pressing on that point validates that the pain is real and that there is an answer. That is so cool!"

Mrs. R returned for another session in about five days. She had not had a headache since the first treatment, but I had her come back one more time. At the third treatment, she still had not had a headache since our first session.

"This is a miracle!" exclaimed Mrs. R. "I should have come here first. My headache problem could have been solved months ago."

"We don't know that, but I too am glad you found your way to my office," I replied.

"Wait, what do you mean we not know that? Nothing else helped, and this treatment approach worked on the very first session. If I would have done this first, the headaches would have disappeared earlier."

One of my students from Chicago, David Fluecke, and I had just talked about this phenomenon over dinner the night before. The discussion was fresh in my mind.

"Clearly, the trigger point work made a tremendous difference in your headaches, however, it is likely that the trigger point therapy would not have been so successful without the good work that the physical therapist and the chiropractor had done before I treated you. We do not know this for sure, but it is likely that they set the stage. All I had to do was finish one last piece of the puzzle. I am not certain, but I would bet that the reason one session alone made such a difference is from the previous good work of other practitioners. Typically, it takes more than one session to effectively treat headaches such as the ones you were having. Since your results lasted, it is likely that the good body mechanics and vertebral mobility you got from them paid off in the end."

Mrs. R thought for a second before nodding in agreement.

"Still, if I would not have come here, I'd still have the headaches today."

"You are probably right," I agreed.

The discussion I had with David Fluecke was replaying in my mind as Mrs. R walked out my door. As David pointed out, it isn't just having the right answer; it is also having the right approach in the right order. There is a time for strengthening, a time for better mechanics, a time for manipulation, and a time for specific soft-tissue work. Choosing the order of therapy could be just as important as the therapy chosen. Trying to strengthen an injured muscle is fruitless, as is manual therapy on a muscle that is truly weak. Like the combination to any lock, the pieces have to be in the right order to unlock it. I don't think enough attention is paid to that. If the results are miraculous, I am hesitant to claim too much credit for PNMT. Conversely, if therapy is failing, it does not devalue the work but may signal the right approach is possibly being done at the wrong time. These are not easy calls to make, but they certainly keep us humble!

The problem with communication ... is the illusion that it has been accomplished.

- George Bernard Shaw

THE ROAD TO SUCCESSFUL THERAPY HAS TWO LANES

She greeted me with enthusiasm in the waiting room; I could tell she was ready for this appointment. Having someone look forward to a session is a wonderful feeling - except in this case.

Earlier that week, I had received several packets of information from her which included some intestinal studies, lab work, and evaluations from several physicians. In essence, there was a colon blockage that was causing severe discomfort. This was a particular blockage I was unfamiliar with, necessitating some research time. The rest of the report contained much information about visceral issues, very little of which was musculoskeletal. Therein began my problem. . .

As she entered the room, she went over the reports with me, clarifying and adding information. She had also seen a PT, who really helped her with some SI joint pain; I know this person and his work is excellent. He seemed to really help her. There did not seem to be any need for me to add to the work he had done.

My dilemma was this: I really had no clue how I was supposed to help this person. Her pelvic floor pain was likely due to the blockage, something that was already scheduled for surgery in a couple of months. If the SI joint was the cause of her pain, my PT friend was already addressing the issue. Where did that leave me?

As I voiced this concern to her, she seemed astonished. I had seen her many times over the years, always for something solvable and with good results. This time though, I wasn't sure it was solvable and when I told her she looked very disappointed at even the suggestion that I was unclear about our goal for today.

"I think that the doctor's assessment that this blockage is the probable source of your pain is correct. I think it seems reasonable that the surgery is necessary. Anything that I could do is very temporary, at best. I don't think that this is a reasonable strategy for you to pursue to deal with this condition."

At this point, tears began welling up in her eyes.

"I am sorry. I have been looking forward to this appointment for weeks. I have been under an extreme amount of stress with this and many other issues in my life; I was so looking forward to having some time to relax."

Now, things were even more unclear to me, plus she was upset and disappointed. Based on what she just said, it seemed like what she wanted was massage for stress reduction. Why though, would she send me over thirty pages of medical reports about this problem if that isn't what she wanted to deal with? Plus, in my clinic, I do not see people for general massage for stress reduction; I only do specific problem solving.

I'd love to tell you that we figured this out and she got what she wanted and needed. In the end, I never did get an answer from her that was clear to me. I kept getting mixed messages about helping this pain and also just having time to relax. After talking about it for about 15 minutes, I was still at a loss and feeling more pressure to do something. I responded by doing general massage that targeted a few areas that *might* have some effect on her pain. She seemed genuinely pleased after the session, so perhaps I gave her what she needed.

In my clinic, about once a month I get a complaint from a client about the work they received from one of my staff. But in the end, the most common reason given is lack of clarity in communication. The day before my experience with this client with pelvic pain, one person complained that the work she received from one of my staff was too specific; she just wanted massage to relax. Yet, in speaking with her, this client admitted that she complained of very specific areas when my therapist did the initial interview. This person just assumed that all massage is pretty general with a slight concentration in one area vs. another. My therapist spent the entire time addressing the areas that this client said needed work. On the other hand, I've had complaints from clients that the massage was not specific enough. In the initial intake interview with the therapist, these same people stated stress reduction and relaxation as the major goal for the massage.

This is not to say that my staff, or myself, have not erred by not delivering what the person really wanted or needed. We have made mistakes and have hopefully learned from them. The road to successful therapy, however, has two lanes. If the client is unclear about the goal, it is nearly impossible for the therapist to be on the correct course. Clarity of communication is the key to ensure therapeutic success.

PAIN, WITH HOPE AT THE END

This morning, I had a very interesting session with Ms. S, a very bright woman with shoulder pain. She has been hurting for months and like many, thought the pain would go away on its own. She stopped playing tennis, then stopped using weights, but the pain did not relent. Finally, she saw a sports medicine doctor, who recommended physical therapy. The exercises recommended were essentially the same ones she had been doing on her own, but she did them diligently. Ten sessions later, her shoulder was worse, not better. In frustration, she sought my services.

"I know my posture isn't great, but I try my best. My physical therapist says to bring my shoulders back, but I mostly forget. I should try harder."

I found this statement a bit surprising, as her carriage and posture seemed hardly a problem in my eyes. In fact, if I had seen her in a social context, I might remark at her fit physique and erect posture in comparison to most everyone else. If her minor shoulder rotation could create pain, then there should be millions of people running around with a lot worse pain than she. That did not make sense.

She was also told by the physical therapist to persevere, to work through the pain. On the other side of the pain was relief, as stated by the PT. This did not match the experience of Ms. S however. No stranger to exercise, she was a college athlete who has always pushed the envelope. This however, felt different.

I palpated her soft tissue, beginning with the most anterior fibers of the upper trapezius. The look on her face told me this was certainly a relevant area to her pain.

"You must tell me if anything is uncomfortable," I said. "I want the treatment to be engaging, but not over-powering."

Her reply was this:

"It is painful, but this is pain with hope at the end."

In all the treatment sessions I have done, no one has ever phrased this concept quite so elegantly. I almost fell off my treatment stool!

In the many lectures I have given on pain, I have often spoken about a unique concept that we as therapists take for granted; that of "good" pain vs. "bad" pain. This concept drives neuroscience people nuts, because pain should be pain, and pain should be avoided. How is it that the nervous system knows that some pain has value, while other pain is just bad? Ms. S somehow knew that the pain from the exercise given to her by the PT was bad. It was not that she was unwilling or lazy; she even overrode her feelings and did them anyway. The results were terrible.

I am sure that there are times when the "good pain" feeling is wrong, but I must say I cannot think of a single instance of that in the clinic.

The lesson here is that we as therapists must listen to our clients. If they strongly feel that what we are doing is helpful, perhaps no single criterion is a stronger validation of possible effectiveness. On the other hand, clients must realize that we cannot know this without their feedback. Clear communication is probably the strongest predictor of therapeutic success.

YES, BUT IT MIGHT HURT

Sometimes when I am teaching, it is fascinating to scan the class, seeing each person looking back at me. Each person has a unique way he /she conduct themselves. Some people eagerly project themselves outward, as if their eyes could leap forward to make a connection. Other people rather pride themselves on creating distance by looking detached, even though they are really paying attention. Others, as you might guess, truly aren't paying attention. For Ms. C, her expression was one of extreme distraction produced by pain.

I would periodically make eye contact with Ms. C, and she would almost immediately cast her gaze downward. As she constantly shuffled in her chair, every five minutes she would punctuate her distress with a long and very audible exhalation. The rest of her classmates were used to this loud sigh and did not respond, or seem to notice. I on the other hand, was not sure how to respond. Each time I glanced at her, she gave a look that said "If you really cared about treating people in pain, you'd be treating me right now."

The next morning, I found a time in class where individual treatment could embellish what we were learning, rather than detract from the class. Ms. C told about her history of back pain, which had begun about seven months earlier. As time went on it became absolutely debilitating, causing her no end of problems, both personally and professionally. (Her pain was at the iliac crest, SI joint, and sometimes, but not always, going down her leg.) It may have begun when she tried to help an elderly person out of a bathtub; a task which there really is no biomechanically efficient way to accomplish. The fact that she had pain going down the leg (past her knee, down to her ankle) pointed to the sciatic nerve, but the episodic nature of the pain seemed like a good sign. She could not climb on the massage table; the transition was too painful. Since effective treatment can easily be done from a chair, I had her stay seated.

Like any treatment, the first key is to decide the hierarchy, what is important and what is not, what is cause and what is effect. In her case, as with anyone who is hyper-reactive, this is not so easy. Everywhere I touched was super sensitive, so much so that just the touch alone was creating a very emphatic and audible reaction from her. The problem was, each area seemed to be incredibly tender, some worse than others. I kept looking for a window of opportunity, but found most of them boarded up. Where to begin?

I decided to pick one area that I knew was probably a player, but not *the* major player. I did not attempt to address what I thought to be the epicenter for fear that she would react too strongly, producing the opposite effect from what I intended. I chose an area that was slightly less reactive, although her reaction was even strong enough to border on making this a risky strategy.

As I touched the area above her iliac crest, she reacted very strongly, but I did not remove my hand from her back. I decided to take a calculated risk and keep my finger right there and allow her system to process the input. Mostly, the tissue would relax, but periodically the pain would increase markedly. I have seen this before with a muscle tear, but never on such large muscles such as the one I was treating. I decided just to hold on, the way a horse trainer just lets the horse know that he or she is not a threat, but is not going to go anywhere either. The treatment space suddenly became a round-pen, where she and I were inside of it and there was nowhere else to go, nowhere to escape. This type of approach is very unusual for me; I cannot remember the last time I have done that with a client.

I followed this strategy with four sensitive areas, the ilio-lumbar ligament, the quadratus lumborum, the gluteus mini-mus, and the piriformis. There was no drastic improvement, merely a slight lessening in the pain.

As she arose from the chair, I could tell that Ms. C was disap-pointed. I am sure that she thought that if I treated her, she would arise from the chair and be amazingly better. It is an intriguing idea, but in real life, improvements are much more a process than an event. After her treatment she walked around the room gingerly. I instructed her to find a comfortable position to sit for the rest of the class but to move as frequently as possible.

The next morning Ms. C was there bright and early. I wanted very much to ask her how she was feeling, but her face told me that she was still in significant pain. Not wanting to distract the class with one case, I did not ask, I just waited.

About one hour into the class, I could not stand the suspense and asked her how she was doing.

"I slept the whole night through for the first time in months" she stated. I was shocked: Her face told me she was still in pain and her periodic audible sighs were about the same as the previous day. If she was better, why didn't she look and sound better? Something seemed incongruous here; she was telling me one thing and revealing another via her behavior. Which was I to believe; what I saw or what I heard?

Later in the day, I decided to readdress the areas we had treated the previous session. I had her in exactly the same position, sitting in a chair. As I palpated the tissue at the top of the iliac crest, she let out the same gasp of pain that she had done the day before. Oddly, what I felt in the tissue actually seemed like improvement (even if I only had a fleeting second to palpate it). The tissue was softer, much less stiff, and I did not feel the nodule-like consistency of the previous day. My assessment, of course, is one thing, what really counts is *her* experience. What I felt in the tissue (slight improvement) did not match with her experience (pronounced reaction to touch).

Moving on, I palpated another area and again, she reacted strongly. Again, the area where I was palpating seemed again much better than the previous day. Moving to the gluteus minimus area, she again responded with pain, which did not match my expectations.

Going back to the iliac crest area, I palpated it one more time and again, she responded strongly.

I had to say something.

"I hate to state the obvious here, but I assume that this is painful, yes?"

The answer I actually got was rather unclear. When I palpated the area again she gasped and jumped. For a second time I asked about pain and the answer was much the same.

"I hate to be harsh, but I need to know if the area I am touching is painful and the answer is simply 'yes' or 'no'. I need to know, is this painful?"

"Well," she said, "it could be."

"Do I take that as a yes or a no? It sounds like a no to me."

"It could be, and has been, very painful," she qualified.

"Yes, I am sure that is true, but I am asking you if it is painful now, right now."

"I guess the answer is no then," she admitted.

"This is extremely important. In order for me to know how best to treat you, I need your feedback. That feedback is vital and I need it to be accurate. When you respond to touch as though it were painful, I cannot tell the difference between your anticipated pain and your real pain. Come to think of it, neither can your brain. . ."

This last comment raised her eyebrows as she struggled to comprehend the exact meaning of the statement.

"Let me explain. In an interesting research study, researchers hooked subjects up to an fMRI machine that registers blood flow to parts of the brain. While the subjects were in the machine, the researchers told the subjects that a very hot object would be placed on their shin. It was indeed hot, enough to cause pain but not tissue damage. Then the researchers told the subjects that the next object would be room temperature and it was. The brain scans between these two experiences were quite different. Various pain centers in the brain lit up with the hot device and were quiet with the room temperature object. Finally, the researchers told the subjects they were going to apply the first device again, the one that was really hot. As the device touched the skin, the brain scan revealed an identical picture to the first scan, with pain centers lighting up massively. The surprising fact is that the device was actually at room temperature. Due to their expectation, the subjects experienced pain. Anticipation of pain created the reality of pain, with no heat needed."

After I finished telling the story, I could see her processing the relevance of this information.

"I'd like to make a deal with you. It is obviously very important for me to know if something is painful. I wish to stay in a comfortable zone for treatment, where you do not recoil in any way against my pressure. I need accurate feedback to do that. Would you only agree to react to real pain rather than anticipated pain?"

What followed was a very different experience. Indeed, she had to restrain her inclination to over-react, but she did a wonderful job at this. I could feel her inhibit inappropriate reactions, pausing to evaluate the experience first. She could much more easily give me feedback; when it was painful I let up. When it wasn't, I continued to examine the tissue carefully.

During the rest of the day, there seemed to be a profound change in Ms. C. She seemed more apt to answer questions in class and take a chance at being wrong. I do not know if I am remembering this correctly, but I do not remember her audible sighs during the afternoon. At the end of the seminar, she stood up and told the class what an epiphany the difference between real pain and anticipated pain was. As she talked, she even made clever jokes, revealing a beautiful smile that her classmates had not seen in months.

PAIN, SHINGLES, AND THE BRAIN

I could see the pain on her face as I greeted J this morning. There is an unmistakable look that someone in pain has, something easy to see but hard to explain. Perhaps it was the look in her eyes or her movements, which were slow and deliberate. Whatever it was, she was in pain and clearly suffering.

After my inquiry, she began to reveal her story. A couple weeks ago, she had noticed a pain in her back at the level of her serratus posterior inferior muscle. The pain slowly began to creep around to the front. It was quite disconcerting and she finally visited a convenient care facility to ascertain the cause of her discomfort. They were unsure and after ruling out several grave causes sent her back home.

When red blotches surfaced, it was very clear that she had an outbreak of shingles. The pain from shingles is a terrible pain, unrelenting and stinging. While it is less disabling than other pains, there is a certain sharpness to the pain that is extremely unpleasant. J had clearly been suffering and was very tired of the pain by the time she arrived in my office.

As I looked at the affected area, I could see that the outbreak had 'healed' quite nicely; more than eighteen days had passed since the beginning of the ordeal. The red spots were barely still visible, but still fully present in J's experience.

"I suppose it was silly for me to come today. I know you can't work on the area that hurts. It is just that I am in so much pain I can hardly think of anything else, and you have always helped me in the past. I was hoping you could do something for me today, but I really don't even know what I am asking you to do."

"Actually, I may be able to help you. Can we explore this?" I asked. "Can you describe your experience of the pain to me?"

J went on to explain how the pain would wash over her. It would come in waves, each time reminding her that the 'devil' was still in the house and wasn't going away anytime soon. She lived in fear for the next wave of pain, and it left her feeling very helpless.

At this point I asked J to describe, in great detail, various aspects of the pain. If it was a color, what color would it be? If it was a metal, what kind of metal would it be? If it was a sound, how would you describe it? As I kept asking questions, J's brain was examining the experience of pain with the cognitive part of her brain, something neuroscientists call higher order processing. Interestingly, higher order processing has a way of diminishing the experience of pain. When the brain is curious about something and is exploring the experience, fear is reduced, and fear is known to increase pain. What research tells us is that the brain needs to view the pain experience as an observer, rather than being overrun with the emotions of pain. According to the International Association for the Study of Pain, pain is an unpleasant sensory *and* emotional experience. The use of "and" rather than "or" is very important. Strategies that move the person from emotion to cognition seem to lessen the experience of pain.

The second strategy I employed was to reduce the stimuli in the vicinity of the outbreak. When there is a problem in one location, the immediate vicinity is also supersensitive to any stimuli. Not only is the periphery of the injury sensitive, it is so abnormally sensitive, it responds to normal stimuli as if it were painful. If you have ever had a burn, you know about this phenomenon. Not only is the site of the burn sensitive, the surrounding area becomes hyper-reactive. The skin around the burn is hypersensitive to touch and to temperature. Neuroscientists call this peripheral sensitization.

Interestingly, I found several areas that harbored trigger points, some of which referred into areas around where J had been having her pain. This phenomenon is right out of the literature and is a known cause of post-shingle pain. Each of these areas was slowly and carefully addressed. It was also important that J experienced pleasure with my touch. To that end, I was careful to make sure that I addressed areas near the shingle outbreak that were not tender. It was very important for her to realize that not everything in that area was sensitive and painful. When in pain, it is easy to generalize the discomfort over a very broad area, blurring the boundaries of injured tissue and healthy tissue. Helping the client reestablish the real boundaries of affected tissue can be a great help in reducing discomfort.

Lastly, I took the time at the end of the session to explain to J the mechanism of the pain and an expected timeline based on the known literature. When the brain understands a time-line, pain is reduced. If I hurt my finger, I fear for my livelihood. If my physician carefully explains exactly what the source of the pain in my finger is, why it happened, and what the expected timeline for healing is, the fear factor (hence pain experience) is much reduced.

When J was leaving the office, she shared that she felt ele-vated and inspired from the intense focus and concentration that we maintained though the session. It was an hour of deep sharing and quiet communication on many levels, a wonder-ful way to begin the day for both of us. At the end of the day, my secretary pulled me aside to say J had called in to report the first pain-free day since her outbreak. Her visit, my first ses-sion, was a good start to the day; her phone call was a great way to end it.

YOU AND I BOTH KNOW

After a very long day seeing of clients in my clinic, I met my wife for a bite to eat and a glass of wine at a local wine bar that has great food. Having been in my community for many years, I often see many people I know when I am out. Tonight was no exception.

Just as our food was coming, a client that I had seen occasionally kept motioning for me to come over to her table. As I did, the conversation quickly went from pleasantries to lateral epicondylitis. (Funny, how that happens!)

As she asked me more questions about the condition, I began to question where this was really coming from. It finally it hit me and I turned to address her husband, who hadn't said a word.

"This isn't about your wife is it? This is about you, correct?"

The husband nodded rather sheepishly, as he admitted that her questions were really about his arm, not hers.

"It's not really that bad, just a little tender," he submitted.

"Just a little tender? Are you kidding me? This morning you dropped the pillow while making the bed! If you can't lift a pillow it is a little more than tender," his wife objected.

That statement was followed by what seemed to be an endless pause, with him staring at her, his wife glancing at me and staring back at her husband. Meanwhile, I just want to get back to my food and a glass of wine, which had just been just been delivered to my table. Her husband, who happens to be a physician, did not know what to say.

"Well, you and I both know why my arm hurts," he replied dismissively.

"You and I both know…" is one of those statements that drive me nuts. I don't think I have ever had someone say "You and I both know…" to me when I actually knew what was coming next. If we both already know, why is the statement that follows almost always a surprise to me?

The husband waited for me to respond, which I resisted. When it was clear that I was not going to take the bait, the husband shared his insight.

"I am sixty-nine years old!" he stated forcefully.

(At this point, I was lamenting that my food was getting cold, my wife was getting annoyed, and my wine was untouched. This was the insight I was waiting for?)

It took me a minute to even concoct a response to such a statement. After a second to ponder, I decided to go a different direction. If I get to play the interlocutor, at least I can have some fun.

"I see. I suppose that makes sense. By the way, which arm is bothering you?" I queried.

"The right one," he replied, in a tone that implied he was pleased that I accepted his explanation and maybe now his wife would stop bugging him about his condition.

Looking him in the eye, I studiously looked at his right arm while nodding in agreement. He seemed to be pleased with this.

"I have one question for you. Just curious, but how old is your left arm?"

I left the question in the air, savoring the look in his eyes when he realized the fallacy of his reasoning.

"Here is my card, call me if you decide to have some treatment on your arm."

I went back to my food; he and his wife sat there, her looking at him, he looking at the floor.

"What was that all about," my wife asked as I returned to the table.

"As you know and I both know, people don't always make sense," I couldn't resist saying. She gave me a look that said "I love you, but sometimes you're a little nuts."

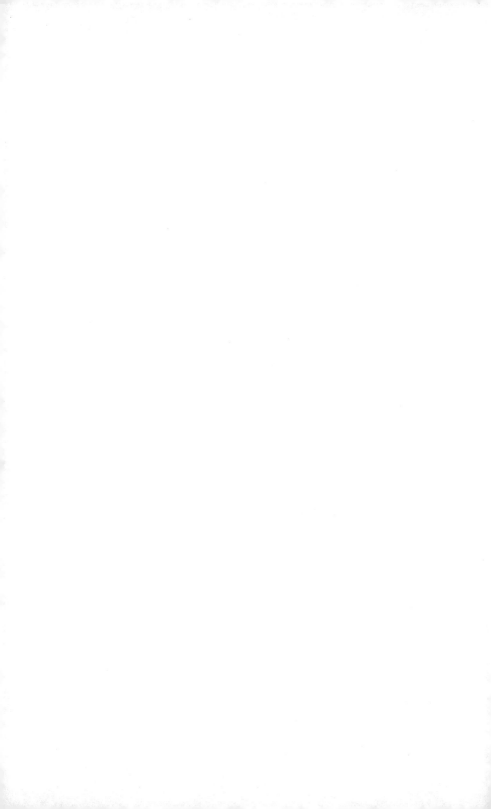

THE FOOTBALL AND THE BALLET SHOE

A young violist or dancer with pain is not treated the same as a star basketball or football player. One gets all the resources, the other is told to redirect their ambition and passion into something else.

She was a charming and intelligent young lady, fourteen years old and in the starring role of a very professionally done ballet performance. This young woman had worked her butt off to get to the leading role in this ballet; the competition was fierce and immensely talented. Opportunities for this kind of role don't come often for people in ballet. There are tons of leagues for kids in sports where multiple kids get the chance to perform. In the arts, the opportunities for really excellent experiences are much less common. There is only one starring role, those positions are much coveted by many talented young dancers.

For my young ballerina, the problem was pain. The stress on the lower extremity in ballet is intense; the demands are unlike any other activity that I know. This young woman had trained for years already, getting serious about dance at age six (she started at age four, but it took two years to get serious!) The hours and dedication she allotted to dance were something we all wish for our children; we want them to find a passion and pursue it. No one was pushing this young dancer, she found her calling and she wanted dance as a career.

As you might expect, when the pain began, she and her family were concerned. Her parents were concerned about their little girl and did not want her to do anything that might worsen the injury. They supported her love of dance, but were concerned for her long-term health first and foremost. Seeing her in pain, they took her to a physician for an exam.

As the young woman described her pain, and the doctor asked more questions about her practice and rehearsal schedule, the prescription was predictable. Essentially, if dancing is causing you pain, then you must take time off from dance for a period of six weeks. This advice was administered after waiting for almost three weeks to get in to see the doctor, during which the family had limited her dancing anyway, not knowing what else to do. Although our young ballerina wasn't happy about it, she did comply by ceasing to dance for almost six weeks. Unfortunately, when she resumed, the pain was right there to greet her. Just to be clear, she did her resumption in an incremental way, so a surge of activity wasn't the cause of her return to pain.

After I finished treating her (the details of which are largely unimportant to the story), I had to rush over to see a star collegiate athlete in a big-time program. The certified athletic trainer had called me that day, and when they ask when you can come, that does not mean some day in the near future, it means what time can you be here *today*. I rushed over to see this athlete as soon as I finished with the dancer, leaving the office in a flurry. As soon as I arrived, the trainer (who is one of the most knowledgeable and sincere I have ever worked with) gave me every detail of this kid's discomfort. He detailed every nuance of the injury: when it started, what the symptoms were, what has been done, what has worked, who has been involved. Before the young man walked in the door, I already had tons of information at my disposal. I knew what questions to ask the athlete and my time could be spent doing meaningful palpatory assessment, that which I do best and the reason they called me in the first place.

After forty-five minutes with this young man, the offending soft-tissue was clearly identified. I had treated him appropriately and the trainer knew how to integrate what I had learned into the daily strength and conditioning that this young man participates in.

As I was driving home, I was struck by the contrast between these two young and talented athletes. If we follow the logic of the first doctor, if the offending activity is the source of your pain, the activity must be ceased for a period of time. Really? In all my years, I have never seen a high profile athlete sidelined in the middle of the season because the medical team thought that six weeks of rest would remedy the problem.

You may be tempted to think that the athlete being pushed back onto the field too early, risking further injury. While this may happen somewhere, I have never seen this at the collegiate level or in the pros. The more valuable and high profile the player, the more incentive there is to do everything right. In my experience, the higher profile the college program, the better the training and support staff. I have been awed by the care and competence I have seen.

In contrast, the dancer received essentially no care at all. Why is that? My young college star played the next game, in fact, did not miss a game all season, and is in excellent shape now. Our dancer was told to give up her dream when the pain returned, something that she and her parents could not accept. Thankfully, one treatment made all the difference. She was able to resume dancing in a matter of days, except now she was far behind in her conditioning, which puts her more at risk for another injury. Waiting was not only a waste of time; it put her at further risk.

It is sad to say, but the difference in allocation of resources is simply attributed to one thing, what we value as a society. A young violist or dancer with pain is not treated the same as a star basketball or football player. One gets all the resources, the other is told to redirect their ambition and passion into something else. How sad.

I could not attend the performance of the ballet to see my young dancer fulfill her dream. I was on the road again, teaching to students in another part of the country. While at dinner that Saturday evening, I happened to glance up at the television in the restaurant to see the young man I had treated in a nationally televised game. While wonderful, it was perhaps even more satisfying to get a text message from a young dancer, thrilled with her performance that evening.

AFTERWORD

It is my sincere hope that reading these narratives has proved to be valuable in deepening your understanding of massage therapy practice. As I reread the stories, I see the face of each client in the story and the valuable lessons I learned in the experience. It is my hope that each story will have an impact for your practice and understanding as it did for mine. In that way, the successes and failures of my singular treatment room are multiplied; helping to advance the understanding of the field of massage therapy. Few feelings are so satisfying.

As I have shared these stories with colleagues and students, many have shared insightful encounters of their own that I found quite inspiring. I could easily see a second volume of Table Lessons that would include narratives from other practitioners. In a field where most therapists are isolated in small treatment rooms, the sharing of insight could be a source of inspiration and shared experience.

If you have client experiences that deepened your understanding and would be willing to share them, please feel free to contact me via email: doug@nmtmidwest.com

ACKNOWLEDGMENTS

This book would not be possible without the support and guidance of so many people who have touched my life, both personally and professionally. Every day, I am aware that I "stand on the shoulders" of all who have come before. This book is a tribute to the rich history of manual therapy practitioners who have pioneered the field.

While I have had many fine teachers in my career, none are greater than a number of brilliant clients who have graced my treatment room over the years. My best education has come through these clients; people who taught me how to think, question, and research. While most people acquire those skills in an academic setting, my thirst for knowledge came later, inspired by the clients who trusted me to help them with muscular discomfort. I will forever be indebted to them and to Champaign, Illinois, the community in which I live. This vibrant community is rich with passionate people and intellectual stimulation.

In addition, I wish to thank my clinic and teaching staff for their support over the years. I cherish the rich conversations about lessons learned from our clinical experiences. Sharing these experiences feeds and inspires me. Thank you also to my clinic manager Debbie Robeck and my daughter Natalie, who is also my seminar administrative assistant, for helping me carve out time in my schedule to write.

I want to thank Leslie Young (editor) and all of the creative staff of Massage and Bodywork magazine for the constant encouragement with this project. Several of the stories in this book have also appeared in a regular column in Massage and Bodywork magazine. If you enjoy these stories, please refer to the magazine for the very latest adventures!

I also wish to thank Carol Leseure for her willingness to read and edit stories. Ever the consummate teacher, she has gently guided me to dive deeper into the joy of writing.

Lastly, and most of all, I wish to thank my wife Janet for her untiring support. She has unceasingly sacrificed to help me pursue the dreams I dream. She is both my inspiration and the one I turn to when the road is difficult.

Douglas Nelson